End of life choices
consensus and controversy

Fiona Randall
Consultant in Palliative Medicine
Royal Bournemouth and Christchurch
Hospitals Foundation Trust
Bournemouth, UK

R. S. Downie
Honorary Professorial Research Fellow
Emeritus Professor of Moral Philosophy
University of Glasgow
Glasgow, UK

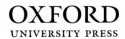

OXFORD
UNIVERSITY PRESS

OXFORD

UNIVERSITY PRESS

Great Clarendon Street, Oxford OX2 6DP

Oxford University Press is a department of the University of Oxford.
It furthers the University's objective of excellence in research, scholarship,
and education by publishing worldwide in

Oxford New York

Auckland Cape Town Dar es Salaam Hong Kong Karachi
Kuala Lumpur Madrid Melbourne Mexico City Nairobi
New Delhi Shanghai Taipei Toronto

With offices in

Argentina Austria Brazil Chile Czech Republic France Greece
Guatemala Hungary Italy Japan Poland Portugal Singapore
South Korea Switzerland Thailand Turkey Ukraine Vietnam

Oxford is a registered trade mark of Oxford University Press
in the UK and in certain other countries

Published in the United States
by Oxford University Press Inc., New York

British Library Cataloguing in Publication Data
Data available

Library of Congress Cataloging-in-Publication-Data

2009932519

Typeset by Cepha Imaging Private Ltd., Bangalore, India
Printed in Great Britain by the MPG Books Group, Bodmin and King's Lynn

ISBN 978-0-19-954733-3

10 9 8 7 6 5 4 3 2 1

Preface

This is a book for all health care professionals who deal with the care of patients towards the ends of their lives—and that is the great majority of hospital clinicians, and all general practitioners and nurses working in primary care. We hope it may also be helpful to those working in specialist palliative care, but it is not a 'palliative care' book. The need for the book has arisen because of the inescapable ethical problems in end of life care, combined with recent initiatives such as the *End of life care strategy* which promotes patient choice in treatment and care at the end of life, and the Mental Capacity Act 2005 which governs decision-making for patients who lack capacity.

These developments are taking place in a changing political and cultural situation in which 'patient choice' has become a central idea. Furthermore, the 'best interests' of patients are perceived to extend beyond the traditional aims of medicine to include psychosocial and spiritual matters, and the relatives of patients are included in the remit of end of life care. These latter changes reflect the pre-existing philosophy of palliative care which is in some ways set apart from mainstream health care; the philosophy attributes to professionals the responsibility for alleviating psychosocial and spiritual problems in patients and their families, and it entails ethical problems which we noted in an earlier work.[1]

Against this complex background, healthcare professionals try to resolve conflicts between values such as enhancing and respecting patient choice on the one hand, and equity and cost-effectiveness on the other. The conflict between promoting the best interests of the patient and those of relatives remains, and is potentially increased by the clinical and political stress on patients dying in the place of their choice. The requirement to give patients information to enable adequately informed and valid consent often conflicts with 'communication skills' advice to disclose information in an individualized way according to patients' wishes regarding content and pace, and also with the desire of both patients and professionals to avoid burdensome decision-making processes at the end of life. So although there is a new vision for end of life care, professionals face an increasingly complex web (or perhaps tangle) of ethical obligations.

In order to provide clinically useful guidance on ethical issues in this complex situation—because hands-on clinicians do not have time to seek out, read and consider all the various national guidance documents relevant to end of life care—we have adopted a particular strategy. We have written a book with two main parts.

In Part 1 we discuss some of the issues of end of life care as they are widely encountered in everyday practice; we draw upon the relevant consensus guidance produced by professional bodies such as the UK General Medical Council and British Medical Association, in accordance with UK law. We note that this guidance stresses the professional responsibility to act only in the patient's 'best interests' at the end of life, assuming the traditional aims of health care and the ethics governing it. In Chapter 1 we show how the concept of consent can accommodate the idea of patient choice as 'choice' is understood in everyday life, and how it has led to the ethically desirable idea of joint decision-making; we then contrast the traditional view of 'choice' with the emerging view of 'consumer choice', drawing out the implications of such a change for end of life care. Overall, Part 1 presents a consensus view on decision-making, including the traditional concepts of best interests and patient choice via consent, focusing particularly on life-prolonging treatment and symptom control, all in the context of current recommendations on care at the end of life.

In Part 2 we discuss some issues in end of life care which are currently controversial. Comprising the first range of controversial issues are those in which the everyday notion of choice is being replaced by the very different idea of 'consumer choice'. Consumer choice is a radical doctrine which challenges the traditional idea of consent and opens the way to other doctrines such as mandatory instigation of advance care planning by professionals, attribution of major (perhaps overriding) importance to achievement of the patient's preferred place of death, and physician-assisted suicide and euthanasia. The second range of controversial issues concerns the widening of the traditional interpretation of 'best interests'. We shall outline the controversial view that 'best interests' should be extended to include psychosocial and spiritual issues, and that the remit of professionals should extend to the best interests of patients' families. Again we try to guide readers through the complexities (and sometimes the contradictions) in current initiatives. We end with some brief conclusions about the criteria which any end of life strategy must satisfy if it is to fulfil the ethically essential aims of humane and realistic health care.

The book has two special features. First, since it fulfils some of the functions of a 'textbook' it is well-referenced to provide a resource for those who wish to follow-up any issue in detail. It has also been written so that each chapter can largely stand alone, but with signposting to other chapters where relevant. Second, we have provided an extensive Appendix in which common ethical theories are outlined. This has been included because some knowledge of ethical theory is required in training courses, and the vocabulary of ethical theory is widespread in current discussions. But textbooks of bioethics or end of life care do not provide systematic expositions of ethical theories, and original sources require more study time than is usually possible for health care professionals. This Appendix can be accessed online at www.oup.com/uk/isbn/9780199547333/

We would also like to express our thanks to the patients, their relatives, and our professional colleagues in health care, who have inspired us to write this book and whose stories have informed our discussion.

Good textbooks should provide guidance through the complexities of clinical practice and current health policies and initiatives; but they should also raise awareness of the pros and cons of current issues. We hope that we have achieved both of these goals, even if in consequence some hackles are raised!

Fiona Randall
R. S. Downie
Spring 2009

Reference

1. Randall F, Downie RS (2006). *The philosophy of palliative care: critique and reconstruction.* Oxford University Press, Oxford.

Contents

List of abbreviations and acronyms

A&E	accident & emergency	NHS	National Health Service
ACP	advance care planning	NICE	National Institute for Health and Clinical Excellence (prior to April 2005 the National Institute for Clinical Excellence)
ADRT	advance refusal of treatment		
APM	Association for Palliative Medicine		
BMA	British Medical Association	OTPM	*Oxford textbook of palliative medicine*, 3rd edn
BMJ	*British Medical Journal*		
CPR	cardiopulmonary resuscitation	PAS	physician-assisted suicide
DoH	Department of Health (UK)	PEG	percutaneous endoscopic gastrostomy
DSM	*Diagnostic and statistical manual of mental disorders*		
		PPC	Preferred Priorities for Care document
EoLCP	End of Life Care Programme		
GMC	General Medical Council	QALY	quality-adjusted life year
GP	general practitioner	WHO	World Health Organization
GSF	Gold Standards Framework		
MRSA	meticillin-resistant *Staphylococcus aureus*		

Introduction

'Patient choice' is not a new idea in traditional end of life care, but the twist it has recently been given in political initiatives and cultural changes is a radical one which may well alter the nature of health care delivery both generally and specifically in end of life situations. Briefly, 'patient choice' is becoming 'consumer choice'. In Chapter 1 we discuss this development and its implications for end of life care. This discussion is the key to opening up the argument of the entire book. In Chapters 2–3 of Part 1 we discuss in more detail the ethics of end of life care delivered in terms of the traditional idea of patient choice and consent, and in Chapters 7–9 of Part 2 we explore the more radical and controversial idea of end of life care delivered in terms of consumer choice.

Going along with the ambiguity in the idea of patient choice there is a second ambiguity, this time in the idea of 'best interests'. Traditionally the doctor would interpret 'best interests' in terms of the three aims of medicine: the prolongation of life, the relief of suffering and the restoration or maintenance of function. In Chapters 2 and 4–6 of Part 1 we interpret 'best interests' in this way. But in Part 2, Chapter 10, we consider whether 'best interests' should be more widely interpreted as 'whole person' or 'holistic' care, or even as 'quality of life'. Indeed, many in palliative care say that the best interests of the relatives should also be considered.

In sum, Part 1 is offering a consensus view of choice (the view which underpins consent) and of 'best interests' interpreted in terms of the three traditional aims of medicine and Part 2 is offering a discussion of current and controversial interpretations of choice and best interests.

Part 1

Patient choice and consent

Consent is a basic concept of both ethics and medical law, so it is not surprising that discussions about consent to treatment are common in the literature of health care ethics. The ethical stress on consent developed from two sources, one legal and one philosophical. The legal source is the law that touching another person without that person's consent is an offence. The philosophical source is the Kantian idea of autonomy; people are self-determining and self-governing (they can exercise free choice) so they must consent to whatever affects them if it has not proceeded directly from their own will. This explanation of the centrality of consent is persuasive as far as it goes, but to understand more deeply the importance of consent in medical practice we must look at the complex way in which the doctrine has continued to develop in clinical decision-making. This will be the concern of Chapter 2.

The discussion and development of the doctrine of consent has gone on *within* medical law and ethics, for example, in the publications of professional bodies such as the UK General Medical Council (GMC) and the British Medical Association (BMA). Parallel to this discussion, however, there has been another debate which takes not consent but 'patient choice' as its central idea. This debate has been conducted to some extent *outside* health care, by politicians and patient groups.[1] In short, it reflects the consumerism of the age.[2] The concept of patient choice is now significantly influencing policies and attitudes in end of life care, particularly in relation to location of care and death.[3] But although 'patient choice' is a central concept in current debate, it is radically ambiguous and therefore it is important at the start of our discussion to examine it closely. It will emerge that there are two important senses of 'choice'. The first sense of choice is the one found in ordinary speech and practice, and indeed, as we said above, it underlies the doctrine of consent as it is found in clinical practice. The second sense derives from the economic structures of the free market economy and it has been imported into health care for political reasons.[4] Health care professionals become understandably confused between the two senses and their impact on the idea of consent. We shall find that this confusion underlies many of the current debates which we shall discuss. We therefore start with the idea of choice in this chapter, and in Chapter 2 take up the more immediately practical professional concerns of consent and its current status in clinical decision-making in end of life care.

1.1 Choice: the traditional concept

The place to begin is ordinary speech, for it is in the stream of life that the concept is most at home. Of course, the concepts of ordinary language are not precise and overlap with related concepts. Thus we shall find that 'choice', as the term is used in everyday contexts, overlaps with concepts such as 'picking' or 'deciding', but we can still make some headway in demarcating the concept of choice. As used in everyday contexts there seem to be four conditions for choice.[5]

First, a choice must in some sense be *free*, in that it is not forced or constrained; the chooser is doing what he or she wants to do. This is not the context in which to open up the philosophical debate on the freedom of the will, but we must at least note that not every philosopher would regard that description of freedom as adequate. After all, it might be said, human desires can be conditioned by many factors. We need not consider drastic matters such as brain washing; everyday conditioning, as from advertisements, clearly affects our wants. Thus, perhaps we may think our choice is free because it expresses what we want, but we cannot choose our wants! This kind of problem we shall leave to philosophers; for present purposes it is adequate to say that the first condition for choice is freedom from external constraints.

Second, a choice requires *alternatives*. You cannot choose for whom you will vote if there is only one candidate. A typical choice situation in everyday life is one in which the chooser surveys a box of chocolates or a holiday brochure. But of course someone might well say 'I cannot make up my mind' and just takes a chocolate, or opens the brochure at random and sticks a finger into the page at which it has opened. These situations are not properly situations of choosing but rather situations of picking. Since language in everyday life is loose (as we said) we might well speak either of choosing or of picking in such contexts. For example, a conjuror might hold open a pack of cards and say equally 'Choose a card', or 'Pick a card'. Hence, if we are going to distinguish choosing from picking we need another condition.

The third condition for choice in everyday contexts is *information*. We cannot be said to be choosing unless we know something about the alternatives; to choose we need information. The information need not be detailed. 'That one is a mint cream' would be enough to count as the choice of a chocolate. In other contexts we would require a great deal of information. If, for example, we intend to choose a car or a computer then we would want to read the booklets and try them out.

But if having considered the alternatives and been given the information we freely choose, then a fourth condition of choice becomes apparent—we take *responsibility* for our choice. If later we complain to our family or friends about what we have chosen they may well say, 'Well, it was your choice.' We are responsible for every decision/action which satisfies the conditions for choice, and if these decisions/actions are significant ones the responsibility is a moral one.

These, then, are the four conditions for choice in everyday speech: freedom, alternatives, information and responsibility. The attentive reader will have noted that they spell out the acronym FAIR! Reflection on these four conditions also provides some hints as to why we regard choice as important. If the conditions were to be expanded it would become clear that they condense the characteristics that make us human, make us persons. J. S. Mill makes the point strongly when he discusses what he calls the 'distinctive endowment of a human being'. He writes that the 'human faculties of perception, judgement, discriminative feeling, mental activity, and even moral preference, are exercised only in making a choice'.[6] If we consider the four conditions of choice we can see how they are developed in Mill's list. Thus to be free, we said, is to express what you feel, granted your perception, informed judgement or mental activity directed at the available alternatives. In other words, making choices expresses our nature as human beings. Hence, we attach great importance to it—from the chocolate box to the ballot box!

This account of choice fits in well with consent to medical treatments for patients with capacity. Our bodies are central to our nature as persons, and medical treatments will affect our bodies. Hence, in end of life care (as in health care generally) it is morally imperative that patients are able to give or withhold consent without coercion (freedom), that they are given alternatives, and that they are given adequate information on their medical conditions and the treatment options offered. (For example, in relation to decisions about further attempts to prolong life in end of life care, patients will often require a great deal of information to enable them to judge whether, in terms of their own priorities, the burdens and risks of the treatments offered exceed the limited benefits.) To consent or to refuse treatments offered is simply to exercise a choice, which satisfies the four conditions mentioned. The professional takes responsibility for selecting and then suggesting the clinically appropriate options which are offered. The patient takes responsibility for choosing between them on the basis of information on the alternative options which have been offered in the context of discussion. The patient's choice so described has become a joint decision with the professional, and it is clear where the responsibility of each lies. This account of patient choice is reflected in national health care guidance, such as a recent consensus statement on the role of the doctor.[7]

If choice is analysed in this way, the way in which the word is used in ordinary contexts, it presents no problems for the concept of consent or for the current consensus on decision-making in medicine. The problem is, however, that there is much more to the current political 'choice agenda' than what is contained in the everyday notion of choice, and therefore in the notion of consent as joint decision-making. The new dimension of choice takes us out of homely contexts and into the arena of consumer choice in a free market.

1.2 **Consumer choice, the free market and the health service**

Some of the conditions for consumer choice sound the same as those for choice in everyday life, but they involve rather more. Moreover, there are additional conditions for consumer choice which are not necessary for the everyday notion. The first of these extra conditions is *competition*. In the free market in which consumers exercise their choices there must be competition of two kinds: among the suppliers of goods and services, and between the consumer and the supplier—the supplier wants to maximize profits and the consumer wants the best product at the cheapest price. The assumption of free marketeers is that competition of both sorts will 'drive up standards' (a favourite phrase) and regulate prices. Now, we can concede that the discipline of the market will (in general) be beneficial for the provision of consumer goods. It is less clear that it is beneficial for the provision of public goods and services such as transport or education. We shall shortly consider its effect on the provision of health services, especially in the context of end of life care.

It should also be noted that effective competition requires advertising. Consumers must know of the existence of goods and services, what they are intended to do, what their advantages are over existing goods and services, and how much they cost. And of course, in addition to providing information, advertisements are designed to tempt the consumer into buying. They appeal to certain aspects of our human nature, such as our desires or anxieties about the future, and they invite us to see ourselves in certain ways, as prudent or attractive. All these matters follow from the concept of competition.

A second condition of choice in a free market is that the supply of goods and services must be regulated for the prevention of *harm* to the consumer. In other words, a free market is not entirely free since a government will interfere to the extent that it will legislate to ensure the safety of the goods and services offered on the market. For example, lead is harmful so toys must not contain it.

Fabrics and furnishings must be non-flammable. A garage will not make certain speed-enhancing alterations to the engine of a teenager's car where that would cause the car to become dangerous. One important aspect of the prevention of harm in the free market concerns the labelling of goods and information on services. The assumption is that consumers are less likely to be harmed if they have adequate information, including warnings, on what they are buying. The extent to which a government is permitted to interfere with the operation of the free market over matters such as food, drink and health is of course contentious – charges of 'nanny state' are liable to be levelled—but the general principle is accepted even in a liberal society based on free market assumptions: that a government may, indeed ought, to regulate the free market to prevent harm to consumers.

A third condition of the free market is that alternative goods and services must be *available*. Now it might be said that the presence of alternatives was a condition of choice in everyday life. This is true and of course the free market model of choice is consistent with choice as it happens in everyday life. But there is an important additional point in this context. When we are offered choice in everyday life, as in a restaurant, the alternatives are in front of us. We choose from what we are offered. But in the free market the alternatives are inexhaustible. If the shop does not have what we want we can go to another shop, or we can order via the internet. In short, the alternatives can be accessed on a worldwide basis. As we shall see, this has an important bearing on the choice agenda in the provision of health services.

Fourth, the consumer in the free market takes *responsibility* for what has been purchased. If you buy it then the responsibility is yours, unless of course the goods are faulty. You have chosen it, and if you have made a bad choice and the item does not fulfil your purposes then you have only yourself to blame. This fourth condition is closely connected with a fifth—the consumer puts his *money* down, or perhaps uses his credit card. The money passes to the supplier and the responsibility for what has been chosen passes to the consumer. These five conditions—competition, harm, alternatives, responsibility, and money (CHARM!)—work well in the free market. In wealthy nations there is a belief in consumer choice, almost as some kind of human right. Governments in the UK and elsewhere have tried to tap into this belief in consumer choice and are trying to model all public services on the consumer choice basis.

1.3 **Some problems with consumerism in end of life care**

The question is: does consumer choice work in a publicly funded health service, especially in the context of end of life care? In answering this question we shall bear in mind that the National Health Service (NHS), for example, has two essential features: it is about the provision of health care, and it is a publicly funded service. Assuming these features, we shall now consider the consequences which logically follow from introducing the consumer choice model into a publicly funded health care system such as the NHS. Many of these consequences have already followed and the question now is whether they are desirable from the ethical point of view, particularly in the context of end of life care.

1.3.i Competition

The first condition was that of competition. Traditionally, competition has not played much part in the operation of the professions (whose activities are often contrasted with those of the market). But at the present time, governments of all political persuasions are stressing competition in the provision of health care. What this means is that hospital Trusts compete with each other, with primary care services, and with independent community providers to acquire or retain business. Moreover, when the government acts to artificially inflame competition by creating financial incentives to develop more providers of community or institutional services, it is in fact subsidizing new providers to make sure they are viable. At the same time patients are encouraged to get the best deal by consulting league tables which claim to show which hospitals are the best and which consultants perform best.[8] League tables give information about factors such as waiting times, meticillin-resistant *Staphylococcus aureus* (MRSA) infection rates, and so on. 'Quality indicators' are shortly to be introduced for end of life care services, including factors such as how many patients actually died in the place of their earlier recorded choice. But there are ethical problems associated with the attempt to introduce competition into the NHS. These concern *equity; economics; quality of care; advertising.*

Equity. In the context of end of life care, very many patients are debilitated and/or elderly and cannot travel. They will therefore be disadvantaged in any competition to travel to the much-vaunted centres of excellence. Second, by definition patients are sick. The sicker they are the less able they are to travel and perhaps the less energy they have to exercise their competitive role in getting the best deal.[9] Patients at the end of life are particularly sick, often have very little energy, and probably do not want to use that limited energy in a competitive struggle to get the best treatment and care, for example from a specialist palliative care service.[10] Third, patients who require urgent care via emergency services are in no position to exercise much choice as they will almost inevitably have to use the nearest service. They cannot 'shop around' to choose what they think is the best community emergency service, or the hospital with the shortest accident & emergency waiting times and the best clinical performance. So it would seem that the very sickest patients, often those receiving end of life care, are those least able to avail themselves of consumer choice. Our concern is for patients at the end of their lives and they are the most vulnerable of all and the least able to compete for attention.

Economic consequences follow from the need to provide enough services to compete with each other. The requirement for multiple providers tends to entail the provision of spare capacity and this is very expensive. If patients are to be cared for at home where this is their choice, independent (and possibly NHS or social services) providers of care will compete for business. The requirements for patients to have a choice between service providers, and for competition between providers, necessarily entails spare capacity in community services.[11] This is especially true in end of life care where patients' need for increased community care is often immediate and unpredictable. Providers of institutional care, such as nursing homes, NHS-funded specialist palliative care units and hospitals, may come to compete for end of life care business where this is funded by the NHS. Both the high cost of having spare capacity, and any subsidy of independent providers (to ensure that they are viable and so providing competition), all using taxpayers' money, or charitable money in the case of hospices, are significant moral problems in the health service. Health care is inevitably rationed in the NHS and resources spent on the creation of competing services are not then available to provide treatment and care.[12] The creation of competition is therefore not cost-effective.

Hospices are expensive to run but they appear cheap as they raise considerable charitable funds to supplement NHS payments.[13,14] The following are currently unclear: how they will be funded in future; what rationing criteria (if any) will be introduced to allocate their very scarce resource; the extent to which patients will access them by exercising choice in a competitive exercise against other patients; and the extent to which they may compete with nursing homes as locations for continuous professional care, but using charitable funds to meet the gap between nursing home and hospice costs. Whilst there are currently no plans in the UK to significantly increase specialist palliative care resources (either NHS or independent via hospice services), specialist services will have to compete with other services. As those other services gear up to compete, then spare capacity is very likely to result.

Quality of care may be jeopardized in a competitive market.[15] The providers are trying to achieve the goal of providing a service at the lowest possible cost in order to attract business from NHS purchasing bodies. This imperative is overwhelmingly likely to compromise the quality of patient care and safety, especially in end of life care which is necessarily labour intensive but where it is that very labour which is essential for high quality care. Government rhetoric speaks of driving up standards of care. But those who work in the service know that the reality is more that the necessity to drive down costs, or at least to provide a service within the national tariff, works contrary to the interests of improving the quality of care and patient safety. This is inescapably the case in labour-intensive end of life care, where unhurried excellent physical care and skilled professional time to provide information, explanation and reassurance are essential for the quality of care. An outcome of reduction in care quality is obviously of great moral importance in the NHS.

Advertising. Competition does not work without advertising. But advertising goes against the whole professional tradition. Imagine commercial breaks saying: 'Come to us for end of life care—because you're worth it!' Currently there is some competition for business between nursing homes, but, as an NHS national tariff for end of life care is introduced, hospitals, NHS specialist palliative care units and hospices are also likely to compete for business. Whereas hospices could use their well-developed fundraising networks for advertising, hospitals and NHS specialist palliative care services may not be permitted to advertise.

Competition in the context of a publicly funded national health service therefore leads to inequity, consumes resources needlessly, is likely to compromise the quality of care, and inevitably leads to advertising which is at best undignified and distasteful (and is currently not allowed by the GMC). As we have illustrated, all of these adverse consequences are likely in end of life care.

1.3.ii Prevention from harm

Turning now to the second condition of the free market as it operates at the present time, we find that there is stress on regulation to prevent harm to the consumer. Suppliers of goods and services are not allowed to put on the market anything which might harm the consumer. This condition has developed in importance since the early days of *laissez-faire* economics. The phrase which once characterized the market—*caveat emptor* (let the buyer look out!)—is hardly applicable at the moment. There is an enormous emphasis on safety, labelling, redress and on everything which might prevent harm to the buyer. Strangely, this condition of the free market seems to be much less emphasized by those who advocate the choice agenda in end of life care. For example, very debilitated patients with incurable cancer may request, and sometimes be given, further chemotherapy on the grounds that they have 'nothing to lose', but they may not be aware and not be told of the very low survival benefit or of the significant risk that the treatment may cause or hasten death.[16] A recent study by the UK National Confidential Enquiry into Patient Outcome and Death (NCEPOD) on the deaths of 600 patients who died within 30 days of chemotherapy concluded that the chemotherapy caused or hastened death in 27% of patients and caused severe toxicity in 43%.[17] It must always be remembered that the basic principle of all health care ethics is: *primum non nocere* ('first do no harm').

Individual health care professionals are now pointing out that 'the customer is not always right',[18] and that what the doctor advises (to promote the patient's wellbeing and to prevent harm from inappropriate treatment) may not be what the patient wants to hear.[19] The philosopher Baroness O'Neill of Bengarve also noted that many patients' choices would harm themselves or others, and are short-sighted, regrettable or irrational.[20]

Another way of looking at the choice agenda in this context emerges if choice is connected with dignity. It has been argued that your dignity requires that you get what you want or (more grandly) that your self-determination is necessarily involved with your dignity.[21] The UK Healthcare Commission regarded choice as necessary for dignity in dying in its report on dignity in care for older people in hospital.[22] Those who take this line may regard physical harm as less important or even unimportant as compared with dignity, and choice (or self-determination) is said to be a necessary component of dignity. Thus they would conclude that it is more important that patients get the treatment or place of care that they choose, even though that choice results in harm in excess of benefit from treatment, or in significantly suboptimal care because of the location chosen. We shall consider the concept of dignity in Section 9.3.

1.3.iii **Alternatives**

The third condition of choice in the free market is that of available alternatives. It may be granted that the idea of alternatives is present in the everyday notion of choice and in the corresponding notion of consent to treatment offered in joint decision-making. But in everyday life (the chocolate box model) and in consent within joint decision-making, the alternatives are presented to patients to choose from, whereas the modern consumer is not similarly constrained. If the shop does not have the model in stock it can be ordered, or we can go to another shop, or to the worldwide market via the Internet. There are no limits to the range of alternatives and it is the consumer who is the dominant figure. This enlarged idea of choice has certainly moved into health care. If one Primary Care Trust or hospital cannot offer the treatment or care regime, then another can. If it is thought to be not cost-effective or not adequately tested then go to the newspapers, write to your MP and in general make a fuss, and it will be made available.

Consumer choice in end of life care would require the NHS to provide all treatments that patients want, regardless of cost-effectiveness—this situation has not quite been reached, but there is general protest, sometimes extending to outrage, if a cancer treatment is judged not to be cost-effective and therefore not made available via the NHS.[23] Consumer choice would also require adequate care to be provided in the setting of the patient's choice—this is currently an aim as we shall see in our discussions on 'preferred place of care' in Chapter 8.

In end of life care, patients are frequently given 'complementary' therapies (such as massage, aromatherapy, reflexology, homeopathy, and relaxation, meditation and visualization training) alongside conventional treatment, despite a lack of evidence of their effectiveness, simply because patients want them. By contrast, there has been little emphasis on giving patients information of satisfactory quality on these therapies.[24] The 2004 UK National Institute for Clinical Excellence guidance on supportive and palliative care for adults with cancer noted with regard to such therapies that 'there is little conventional evidence on the effectiveness of these therapies for the relief of pain, anxiety or distress, or for improving quality of life.' Yet it recommended that commissioners of care should make complementary services 'available for particular groups of patients, ensuring equal access for all patients meeting the relevant criteria', on the grounds that patients wanted such therapies.[25]

1.3.iv Responsibility

If a consumer obtains the desired goods then the consumer is responsible for making a personal choice—others cannot be blamed if the consumer does not like the goods when unwrapped. Provided the goods purchased 'do what it says on the tin' then *caveat emptor*! A sympathetic retailer might, for reasons of good will, take the goods back but is not legally or morally obliged to do so. By contrast, in health care the responsibility for treatment or care provided remains with the professional in charge. There are a few situations when patients take responsibility. If patients discharge themselves from hospital against professional advice, they will be asked to sign a form explaining that they are taking responsibility for leaving. If the choice agenda develops for treatment then the use of such forms would surely need to become more common. It would be quite unjust if professionals had to take responsibility for choices made against professional advice, whether those choices entailed receipt of treatment or its refusal.

Members of the public taking part in a GMC consultation clearly realized the link between patient choice and patient responsibility; they decided that patients should be entitled to demand treatment against their doctors' wishes, so long as the patients took explicit responsibility for the consequences.[26] Although it is reassuring to note that the public did not think that doctors should be held responsible for the effects of treatment given against their advice, they clearly did not recognize that the doctor cannot escape moral (or currently legal) responsibility for giving the treatment.

1.3.v **Money**

There is a final condition of choice in a consumer society. The consumer may purchase goods against the advice of the retailer—as we say, 'It is your choice.' Not only must the consumer take responsibility for the purchase but he must also put his money down. Now in a publicly funded health service, such as the NHS, the treatment is free at the point of delivery. The patient does not put his money down. It is the taxpayer who does. How fair is it then that the taxpayer should be footing the bill for treatments which are not professionally thought to be appropriate in a given case, or which are judged by national criteria to be not cost-effective, simply because the patient chooses them?[27] It would be perfectly possible to run a system of health care in which the patient pays up front for treatment. Would a patient then demand treatment which was not recommended? At the moment we seem to be in an uneasy position whereby a patient can choose almost anything that he or she wants by way of treatment, but the taxpayer pays. Moreover, since the health budget is limited, this will in effect mean that some other patients will not get treatments which in their case would be beneficial. The obvious example of this problem is palliative treatments for cancer which are not cost-effective.

In end of life care the costs of actual physical care are also significant, partly because it is necessarily labour intensive. Consumer choice would require that patients received an adequate package of care in the setting of their choice. If that choice is home then one-to-one care, 24 hours per day, would be required for many months for those highly dependent patients without family carers who have illnesses such as end-stage dementia or degenerative neurological diseases. The costs to the taxpayer would be enormous, and much greater than the alternative of institutional care.

1.4 **Implications of a system for end of life care based on consumerism**

Finally we shall consider the implications of consumer choice in end of life care. What would a true consumerist health care system be like? It would have four implications of major importance in the ethics of health care at the end of life.

1.4.i **Consent**

In the traditional model the doctor offers only those options believed to have realistic potential for achieving net benefit and the patient consents to or refuses what the doctor offers. By contrast, in the consumer model the patient is requiring the doctor to provide what the patient wants and the patient is then not consenting to the treatment but authorising the doctor to carry it out.

For example, patients could seek information on the Internet about various pain killers (including opiates) and then expect that the doctor would prescribe the drug of the patient's choice, perhaps even beginning at a dose the patient chooses. Or the patient, having sought information, might expect the doctor to provide a treatment which in some cases might have realistic potential to prolong life but which in the patient's case was overwhelmingly likely to yield net harms rather than benefit—in a consumerist model the doctor (and other involved professionals) would provide the treatment even if it was judged clinically inappropriate for that patient. An example would be palliative chemotherapy for non-small cell lung carcinoma where the patient had a poor performance status and cerebral metastases. Or a patient might request a heart transplant because of worsening heart failure, and then expect that this would be carried out even if the patient did not meet clinical criteria for a transplant. Or a patient overwhelmed with hopelessness after receiving a diagnosis of a terminal illness might request a prescription for a lethal dose of medication for the purposes of suicide, and expect that the doctor and pharmacist would comply with the prescription.

In the consumerist system the doctor has become merely the agent of the patient. It might be argued that the doctor could conscientiously object to carrying out a treatment the patient requested when the doctor judged that the foreseen harms and risks were very likely to exceed the benefits. But note the extraordinary paradox: in this situation the *doctor* has become the one who consents to (provide) the treatment and the patient the one who authorizes!

1.4.ii **The concept of a profession**

A doctor or nurse would become simply a purveyor of goods and services, like a baker or a jeweller, or a shop assistant. A doctor would not be required to have the values of the profession, or to exercise professional judgement. For example, the Royal College of Physicians' report on professionalism expects doctors to have the qualities of integrity, compassion, altruism, continuous improvement, excellence, working in partnership with members of the wider health care team.[28] The qualities of compassion, integrity and working in partnership are all particularly needed in end of life care, and are essential when the patient lacks capacity so is less able to exercise the consumer function. But these qualities do not feature in the consumer choice model and indeed they are out of place in that model. Raymond Tallis, representing the College working party, noted that intensifying consumerism has resulted in rising patient expectation which does not match what can be delivered in routine practice; much dissatisfaction has resulted plus increasingly intrusive policies that prescribe medical practice ever more closely, without narrowing the apparent gap between what some patients want and what they get.[29]

A report on medical professionalism by an independent body, the King's Fund, noted fears that consumerism as it equates to consumer choice would lead to patients insisting on a personal choice irrespective of any advice from a doctor. They concluded that the growth of consumerism could pose a threat to medical professionalism.[30]

The consumer model is particularly inappropriate in end of life care, where the need for the qualities of compassion, integrity and working in partnership should be stressed, not negated. Consumerism has its own ethics and responsibilities, but they are quite different from those of professionalism. This can be seen clearly if we contrast professional and commercial motivation.

1.4.iii **Motivation**

Perhaps the most serious consequence of implementing consumer choice in a publicly funded and organized end of life care system is that it would lead to a change in motivation among the professionals. In the consumer choice model the provider of the service is motivated less by a desire to improve the overall welfare of the consumer than to provide goods and services which will satisfy the consumer's requirements at the lowest possible cost to the provider, thus achieving a financially acceptable profit margin.

Indeed, the situation is worse than that. The wages of many sales assistants are at least partly based on commission. In a similar way the salaries of general practitioners (GPs) at present are at least partly based on their success in investigating/treating patients to achieve a target coverage specified by the government. But the GMC stipulates that doctors have a duty to 'make the health of your patient your first concern' in order to justify the trust patients put in them.[31] Trust is the foundation of the doctor–patient relationship and patients still believe that their doctors are uniquely concerned with their health. Will it continue to be true that doctors 'are making the care of their patients their first concern' when patients are seen to be a means of gaining more income for GPs when they achieve an end of life care target?[32,33] GPs have expressed concern that payment for achieving targets is demotivating, damages the confidence of doctors in making judgements based on the best interests of the individual, and has caused us to arrive at a point where the very nature and content of the doctor–patient encounter is prescribed by the state.[34] Will it continue to be true that hospice or hospital staff make the care of patients their first concern when patients admitted to a hospice or Foundation Hospital Trust are seen to be a means of making a profit/remaining financially viable, thus creating a powerful incentive for professionals to encourage patients at the end of life to be admitted to these facilities?

Dr Iona Heath, a GP with 30 years of experience, noted the impact of consumerism on health care under the heading 'Market values and the destruction of vocation':

> By introducing market values into the transaction of health care and turning patients into consumers, while at the same time putting strict limits on the resources available, the Government has trapped health care workers in the credibility gap between rhetoric and reality. Charters offer a superficial vision of quality which has everything to do with being a consumer but very little to do with the needs, priorities and responsibilities of being a patient.
>
> For us as health workers, every component of health care appears now to have its price—we are exhorted to consider the financial implications of our every action. Not surprisingly this has led us in our turn to consider the financial value attributed to our work and this has resulted in an attrition of vocation . . . . Patients are turned into consumers and given rising expectations of what they have a right to expect, doctors are turned into purveyors of a commodity rather than members of a vocational profession providing a public service.[35]

The damage that can be done by consumerism, market values, and associated performance indicators with financial rewards has been noted outside the medical profession. Baroness O'Neill noted that whereas some performance indicators might provide poor measures of complex activities (such as end of life care), others are more damaging in health care in that they create perverse incentives for institutions and professionals and so risk worsening rather than improving medical practice.[36]

1.4.iv The art of dying lost by consumerism

Consumerism does not merely give patients the right to make choices, it actually forces them to make choices. Thus all patients must decide how and where they would like to be cared for, and may be expected to indicate their treatment and location preferences in advance. Every patient with capacity, however debilitated, anxious and exhausted, must make a large number of decisions about treatment and care. In a sense, every individual has to work out for himself how best to get through the final illness and the process of dying. David Clark, a medical sociologist, notes that in modern Western culture one of six elements of a 'good death' is death according to personal preference and in a manner that resonates with the person's individuality.[37] But this implies that each person has to confront death and then work out his own preferences.

This health care culture may not actually be the best for patients—so much decision-making about how to die may be burdensome. It has been noted that choice overload can cause the debilitating effects of bewilderment and high levels of anxiety and stress.[38]

There is some evidence to suggest that patients in developing countries and living in traditional communities have fewer unmet psychosocial needs than patients in developed countries.[39] The reason may be that in those other cultures there is an acceptance of dying and a shared community knowledge of 'how it is done' and how families, friends and patients can support each other in the process. In other words, there is an 'art of dying'. In consumerism there could be no such art embedded in the community, as every person has to work out his own attitudes and values and then make a succession of choices. Quoting a statement by Michael Ignatieff, Iona Heath eloquently expresses the adverse effect of the replacement of this art of dying by a culture of individual choice:

> Most other cultures, including many primitive ones whom we have subjugated to our reason and our technology, enfold their members in an art of dying as in an art of living. But we have left these awesome tasks of culture to private choice.[40]

Having noted these four consequences, the ethical problem of consumerism in the NHS generally, and in end of life care in particular, becomes clear. It will predictably weaken the unique trust that patients should be able to place in their health care professionals. Furthermore, it could actually destroy the concept of medicine as a profession, and certainly as a vocation. When patients are at the end of their lives, and often at their most vulnerable, they have great need for their doctors (and other professionals) to act according to traditional professional values. Lastly, by the inescapable move from a right to choose to a duty to choose, it risks adding to the stresses at the end of life, and it also precludes patients and families from having the security of knowing 'how it is done'.

1.5 **The roots of the choice agenda**

How has the consumer choice agenda risen to such prominence in the doctor–patient relationship? There are several strands to the explanation—philosophical, medical, and cultural.

First, from the *philosophical* point of view the choice agenda has come about through a misunderstanding of Kant's concept of the autonomy of the will. Kant argued that the essence of a person—what gave them dignity—was their ability to be self-determining and self-governing. In particular he stressed the importance of being self-governing, or of being able to act in terms of laws valid for all because they were based on reason. He saw the human will, or decision-making ability, as the source of these rational laws and policies. Other living creatures are pushed around by the causality of their desires and instincts, but human beings have the ability to stand back from the promptings of desire and act in rational ways. It is for the possession of this ability—unique among living creatures—that they are worthy of respect. Just as we might respect or honour a great statesman (e.g. Martin Luther King) or a great artistic genius (e.g. Shakespeare) for his gifts, so (Kant argued) should we respect (or 'reverence' he sometimes says) all persons for their unique capacity to be self-governing.[41]

Unfortunately, as Kant's ideas were taken up by health care ethicists they were distorted. The autonomy of the will was seen merely as the ability to be self-determining, which in turn became the ability to choose whatever one wants. The idea of rational laws valid for all people was lost. Hence, to 'respect' autonomy became just doing what the patient wants. There is a major moral difference between Kant's concept of autonomy and the current concept of the primacy of getting what you choose. Moreover, since Kant thought that autonomy and human dignity were necessarily connected, it was an easy misunderstanding to say that respecting patients' dignity is simply doing what they want or choose (see Section 9.3).

More recently the interpretation of autonomy as the ability to choose, coupled with an imperative to respect such autonomy, has been noted by Baroness O'Neill to be an undesirable basis for health care ethics:

> On the simplest and weakest view, *individual autonomy* is only a matter of individual choice, and respect for autonomy only a matter of respecting individual choice. Respect for individual choice is likely to be morally important, but it is not (*pace* libertarians) likely to be the only thing that is morally important .... An unconditional respect for *individual autonomy* is a highly selective and incomplete basis for ethics or for medical ethics.[42]

It should also be noted that consumerism leads to an idea of the human self very different from that found in the main philosophical tradition. We have already noted (Section 1.1) that J. S. Mill speaks of a natural human endowment which is expressed through choice. He writes that the 'human faculties of perception, judgement, discriminative feeling, mental activity, and even moral preference, are exercised only in making a choice.'[43] In other words, he is assuming (along with the main philosophical tradition) that there is an essential self which can express itself through choice. And other concepts such as dignity will also depend on aspects of that essential self. But in terms of the philosophy of consumerism, the self consists simply in the ability to express preferences through choice. Other concepts are reduced to this. Thus some ethicists make the extraordinary claim that it an affront to patients' dignity if they do not get what they choose.[44]

Second, the choice agenda received an impetus from the *medical idea* of 'patient-centredness'. This term has been in vogue for some years but it tends to have several meanings.[45] In one sense it is simply a truism: the whole aim of medical practice is to benefit the patient. But during the twentieth century the charge of paternalism was directed at medical practice. There was a widespread view that treatment was directed at what the doctor considered to be in the best interests of the patient and that the patient had no input into the treatment decisions. Patient-centredness can therefore be seen also as a reaction against this sort of paternalism. A third sense of patient-centredness is more problematic. Behind the slogan there was the idea that what mattered were the interests of patients rather than any consideration of resources or organizational issues for systems such as hospitals and GP practices. The trouble with this sense, however, is that its proponents ignore two inconvenient facts: that any health budget must have limits, and that a doctor or a hospital has more than one patient. Hence, issues of equity and 'opportunity costs' for other patients inevitably arise. Granted the assumption of scarcity of resources in the health service, providing services for one patient necessarily means depriving another of the benefit of that resource—this is termed the opportunity cost. If 'patient-centredness' means that resources should be inequitably centred on a given patient or population of patients according to their 'choices' then the idea must be rejected.

The third root of the choice agenda—which we are calling *cultural*—is the tap root. It derives its strength from the rise of consumerism and more generally from the rhetoric of individual rights. The viability of Western liberal democracies depends on the economics of the free market economy. But if consumerism is the dominant idea of market democracies it is not surprising if consumerist ideas spread to health care provision, including end of life care. Moreover, consumerism depends on the recognition of individual rights. Hence, consumerism in health care goes along with the assertion of individual rights, and even gives rise to implausible rights such as a 'right to health' or a right to assisted suicide by health care professionals (see Chapter 9). In other words, patients as consumers have a right to choose. The development of the choice agenda has therefore been inevitable, even to the extent that it now pervades end of life care.

1.6 **Conclusions**

1) The idea of patient choice can exist comfortably in the consensus view of health care. In that context, a stress on choice is simply a stress on the patient's right to choose between treatment options offered in the process of joint decision-making, and so to consent to or to refuse those options.

2) Over the last two decades a much more radical idea of patient choice has developed in terms of which patients are regarded as consumers of health care and their choices are construed in terms of a free market economy.

3) Such a view of patient choice has serious implications for the key ideas of consent, resources, equity, and the whole idea of a profession with the values which have traditionally been associated with it. These implications are particularly important in end of life care.

4) It may be possible to provide an end of life care service run on consumerist lines but this would involve extreme deviations from the values of a publicly funded health service.

References

1. Department of Health (2005). *Now I feel tall.* DoH, London, p. 2.
2. Delamothe T (2008). A comprehensive service. *BMJ* **336**:1344–5.
3. Department of Health (2008). *End of life care strategy.* DoH, London, p. 28.
4. Goodrich J, Cornwell J (2008). *Seeing the person in the patient.* The King's Fund, London, p. 25.
5. Downie RS, Randall F (2007). Choice and responsibility in the NHS. *Clin Med* **8**:182–5.
6. Mill JS [1859] (1962). *On liberty.* Collins, London, p. 187.
7. Medical Schools Council (2008). *Consensus statement on the role of the doctor: past, present and future.* Available at: http://www.medschools.ac.uk/documents/FinalconsensusstatementontheRoleoftheDoctor.doc (accessed on 20.01.2009).
8. O'Neill O (2004). Accountability, trust and informed consent in medical practice and research. *Clin Med* **4**:269–76.
9. Woolhandler S, Himmelstein D (2007). Competition in a publicly funded healthcare system. *BMJ* **335**:1126–9.
10. Bate P, Robert G (2005). Choice: more can mean less. *BMJ* **331**:1488–9.
11. Ham C (2008). Competition and integration in the English National Health Service. *BMJ* **336**:805–7.
12. Radcliffe M (2004). Choice cuts. *BMA News*, Saturday 28 August, pp. 6–7.
13. Department of Health, op. cit. (ref. 3), p. 151.
14. Armitage M, Mungall I (2007). Palliative care services: meeting the needs of patients. *Clin Med* **7**:436–8.
15. Bevan B (2008). Is choice working for patients in the English NHS? *BMJ* **337**:a935.
16. Munday DF, Maher EJ (2008). Informed consent and palliative chemotherapy. *BMJ* **337**:a868.
17. Mayor S (2008). UK audit highlights need for caution with chemotherapy in very sick patients. *BMJ* **337**:a2498.
18. Spence D (2008). The revalidation question. *BMJ* **337**:a1353.
19. Colman R (2007). To care for patients' wellbeing. *BMJ* **335**:1169.
20. O'Neill, op. cit. (ref. 8), p. 273.

21. Downie J (2004). Unilateral withholding and withdrawal of potentially life-sustaining treatment: a violation of dignity under the law of Canada. *Journal of Palliative Care* **20**:143–9.

22. Commission for Healthcare Audit and Inspection (2007). *Caring for dignity*. CHAI, London, p. 27.

23. Hawkes N (2008). Why is the press so nasty to NICE? *BMJ* **337**:a1906.

24. Ernst E (2006). We must give patients the evidence on complementary therapies. *BMJ* **333**:308.

25. National Institute for Clinical Excellence (2004). *Improving supportive and palliative care for adults with cancer*. NICE, London, pp. 148–51.

26. General Medical Council (2005). Two sides to every story. *GMC Today*, Issue 05, pp. 8–9.

27. Delamothe T (2008). A centrally funded health service, free at the point of delivery. *BMJ* **336**:1410–12.

28. Royal College of Physicians (2005). *Doctors in society: medical professionalism in a changing world*. Report of a Working Party of the Royal College of Physicians of London, London.

29. Tallis RC (2006). Doctors in society: medical professionalism in a changing world. *Clin Med* **6**:7–12.

30. The King's Fund (2008). *Understanding doctors: harnessing professionalism*. The King's Fund, London, pp. 17–18.

31. General Medical Council (2006). *Good medical practice*. GMC, London, p. 1.

32. Spence D (2008). Lay your money down. *BMJ* **337**:a2619.

33. Delamothe T (2008). A good QOFfing whine. *BMJ* **337**:a2632.

34. Mangin D, Toop L (2007). The quality and outcomes framework: what have you done to yourselves? *British Journal of General Practice* **57**(539):435–7.

35. Heath I (2008). *Matters of life and death*. Radcliffe, Oxford, pp. 94–5.

36. O'Neill, op. cit. (ref. 8), p. 271.

37. Clark D (2002). Between hope and acceptance: the medicalisation of dying. *BMJ* **324**:905–7.

38. Bate P, Robert G (2005). Choice: more can mean less. *BMJ* **331**:1488–9.

39. Murray SA, Grant E, Grant A, Kendall M (2003). Dying from cancer in developed and developing countries: lessons from two qualitative interview studies of patients and their carers. *BMJ* **326**:368.

40. Ignatieff M (1984). *The needs of strangers*. Vintage, London, pp. 76–7.

41. Kant I [1785] (1948). *Groundwork of the metaphysic of morals*. Hutchinson's University Library, London, pp. 100–108.

42. O'Neill, op. cit. (ref. 8), p. 273.

43. Mill, op. cit. (ref. 6), p. 187.

44. Downie, op. cit. (ref. 21), pp. 143–9.

45. Goodrich, Cornwell, op. cit. (ref. 4), pp. 18–29.

2

Choice and best interests: clinical decision-making in end of life care

In this chapter we shall focus on the stages in clinical decision-making in end of life care, drawing attention to issues of particular importance in this context. (The same stages are followed in decision-making in any domain of health care.) This analysis will include the distinctions between the process for patients who have capacity and those who lack it, taking in the ethically important assessment of capacity. In Chapter 3 we shall examine three logical distinctions which are integral to the process of decision-making in end of life care: the distinctions between intended and foreseen consequences, acts and omissions, and killing and letting die. An understanding of these distinctions is essential in the clinical practice of end of life care, and is also necessary to defend decision-making against criticism from an ethical point of view.

It is possible to identify four distinct stages or elements in decision-making in end of life care:

1) Understanding the clinical problem.

2) Selecting the range of treatment options which offer prospect of net benefit.

3) Assessing the patient's capacity for this decision if there is any reason to doubt it.

4) Making the final decision.

In the case of the last stage, making the final decision, a process of 'consent as shared decision-making' is used with patients who have capacity for the decision. For those who lack capacity, a different decision-making process, which focuses primarily on the patient's best interests, is followed (unless the patient has made an advance decision to refuse the treatment or has appointed a lasting power of attorney with authority for the decision in question).

There is some overlap in the timing of these stages in end of life care, nevertheless it is helpful to consider them as separate elements in the process. Practising clinicians tend to follow this process almost subconsciously, but it is necessary to analyse each stage in order to identify and discuss aspects which are of particular ethical importance in end of life care.

2.1 **Understanding the clinical problem**

The essential first stage in decision-making involves knowing what information is relevant, gathering that information, and assimilating it so that it can be carefully considered. Sometimes we fail to make a good decision because we do not appreciate that some specific piece of information is relevant, and therefore either fail to obtain it or fail to use it in the decision. A great deal of knowledge is sometimes important in even apparently simple decisions.

Medicine has three traditional aims: the alleviation of suffering, the prolongation of life, and the restoration or maintenance of function. These three aims are often summarized by saying that health care professionals should pursue the best interests of their patients via diagnosis and treatment. In end of life care we will know the diagnosis, but knowledge about prognosis, relevant further investigations, and the benefits, harms and risks of treatment options is obviously required and is part of our basic professional expertise. Whereas the benefits of end of life care derive from success in achieving the aims of medicine, inevitably there are harms and risks. By harms we mean side-effects and the burdens of undergoing the treatment, and by risks we mean the things that can go wrong. We also require some knowledge about the patient's social background including present social circumstances. All of this knowledge is broadly scientific, and is about similarities between illnesses, and between patients in social settings.

Whereas the *science* of end of life care is about similarities, the *art* of such care lies in addressing the particularities or uniqueness of each patient's situation. So this first stage of decision-making also requires us to gather information and understanding about this particular situation, relating both to this illness and this patient. A certain amount of such knowledge is derived from the case history, which is about how the illness developed and progressed in this patient. But another component in the art requires imaginative and intuitive insight into the meaning of this illness for this person.[1] This includes trying to ascertain the patient's understanding of the illness, the outcomes that the patient seeks, and their own opinion regarding priorities. It also includes trying to ascertain outcomes or adverse events that this patient is keen to avoid. The General Medical Council (GMC), in its guidance on consent, stresses the importance of trying to ascertain patients' 'views, experience and knowledge' regarding their condition.[2] Part of the art of gaining this information is to encourage patients to express their understanding and views about their illness, plus their priorities, while avoiding intrusive personal questioning or pressure to disclose that which they would prefer to keep private.

It is obvious that gaining insight into the patient's perceptions of the illness and priorities requires time (a scarce resource in hospital and primary care clinics), and a warm and friendly listening manner on behalf of the professional. These requirements are acknowledged in the professional literature about decision-making,[3] but they tend to be confused with notions of 'respect' and 'dignity'.[4] Such conceptual confusion makes the doctor–patient conversation appear unnecessarily complex from an ethical perspective. It also tends to give health care professionals the mistaken idea that they need special training to enable them to have a mutually helpful discussion with a patient!

If the patient lacks capacity, due to a coexisting illness such as dementia or due to the pathology of the terminal illness itself, the professional should still seek some individualized understanding of the patient's story, together with some idea of what his or her priorities might have been for the current circumstances. Patients who lack capacity might still be able to express wishes and make known those experiences which they find distressing. Discussion with appropriate family members or friends is also necessary, plus careful scrutiny of any advance statement the patient may have made. (Advance statements are discussed in Chapter 7, and advance statements relevant to location of care in Chapter 8—both are controversial.) The practical difficulties of eliciting information about the patient's wishes, and feelings, beliefs and values from the patient's family and friends are well known to those who have tried. Relatives often find it very difficult or impossible to judge how the patient would have viewed the situation, or are reluctant to take responsibility for that judgement. Gentle encouragement is often needed. We discuss this issue further in Section 2.5, on 'making the final decision' for patients who lack capacity.

We describe this task as a single stage because patients usually disclose the more personal aspects of their story alongside an account of treatment to date and current symptoms. Furthermore, all the information has to be considered as a whole.

2.2 Selecting the treatment options which offer a prospect of net benefit

We have already noted that in health care generally, and in end of life care, the patient's best interests are seen in terms of pursuing the three traditional aims of health care, namely alleviation of suffering due to illness, restoration or maintenance of function, and prolongation of life. So benefit is construed as whatever will achieve these aims via health care interventions. Whether the patient has capacity or not for the decision in question, the professional has to decide what treatment options would offer a reasonable prospect of overall benefit, following comparison of the potential benefits with the harms and risks that the treatment entails. The GMC summarizes this selection process in its guidance on consent:

> The doctor uses specialist knowledge and experience and clinical judgement, and the patient's views and understanding of their condition, to identify which investigations or treatments are likely to result in overall benefit for the patient.[5]

The GMC gives more explicit guidance about this professional role in its guidance on withholding and withdrawing life-prolonging treatment. The principles expressed in that guidance are especially relevant in end of life care:

> Doctors have an ethical obligation to show respect for human life; protect the health of their patients; and to make their patients' best interests their first concern. This means offering those treatments where the possible benefits outweigh any burdens or risks associated with the treatment, and avoiding those treatments where there is no net benefit to the patient.[6]

It is sometimes helpful to consider the four possible patterns of benefit to harm and risk which would offer net benefit. Treatments falling into any of these four categories should be selected for offer to patients with capacity, and consideration for patients who lack capacity. So treatment options selected are those which offer the following:

1) Good or reasonable hope of benefit with low or moderate harms or risks.

2) Good or reasonable hope of benefit with significant harms or risks.

3) Low likelihood of benefit but with low or moderate harms or risks.

4) Small chance of a major benefit, such as cure, much improved comfort or function, or very significant prolongation of life, even if the associated harms and risks are great, since some people would wish to accept significant harms and risks for a small chance of a major benefit.

The professional should *not* offer patients with capacity, or consider for patients lacking capacity, treatment options which:
may have a minimal benefit in some cases but which the professionals judge *in this case* would entail overwhelming harms/risks in comparison to the small chance of benefit.

Examples of such treatments that should not be offered are: attempted cardiopulmonary resuscitation where there is no realistic prospect of success; palliative chemotherapy where there is a very low likelihood of disease response (10–20%) and the patient's performance status is 3–4 so that there is a very high likelihood of severe side-effects and risk of death through neutropenic sepsis in an already debilitated patient; insertion of a gastrostomy feeding tube percutaneously in a patient with motor neurone disease, severely compromised and deteriorating respiratory function, and a significant risk of death during the procedure.

Categories 2–4 above are included on the grounds that doctors should not make assumptions about how the patient would weigh up the relative benefits to harms and risks—patients vary in the weight they attach to different sorts of benefit, harm and risk. The GMC instructs that doctors should not make assumptions about the clinical or other factors a patient might consider significant,[7] and that they must not make assumptions about a patient's understanding of risk or about the importance they attach to different outcomes.[8] Writers coming from an academic background in health care ethics and management have made similar observations, stressing that selection of the best treatment options for each patient requires the contribution of both patient and doctor,[9,10] and that where the balance of benefit to harm and risk is uncertain the decision should be guided by the patient's preferences.[11]

Whereas it is possible to justify an offer of any treatment in categories 1–4 above, it is clearly impracticable, unreasonable, burdensome and possibly stressful for patients to be presented with long lists of options plus information about their benefits, harms and risks.[12] In the context of end of life care there are usually only a few options, and professionals begin by offering those which they think are the best for that patient. Other options are considered if, in the process of joint decision-making, it emerges that those initially presented are not optimal for that patient. A plan can be negotiated which is mutually acceptable to doctor and patient, though this may require giving patients more time and information, which can be difficult in end of life care if the patient is debilitated and becoming more exhausted physically and mentally.[13]

Selection of treatment options in end of life care is difficult; it requires the exercise of clinical judgement because of uncertainties and the difficulty of applying evidence to the situation of the particular patient. Slavishly following treatment 'guidelines' is unlikely to result in the best selection for the patient. This problem is well known in general practice. The general practitioner Des Spence has written an impassioned plea against it:

> Evidence is treated like solid bricks rather than the shanty corrugated iron that it is. This is a slow garrote of medical judgement. Doctors are under the constant spectre of litigation, haunted by the phrase "Did you follow the guideline, doctor?" So discretion, once the keystone of the medical profession, is dead . . . . I often want to ignore the guidelines, for they don't reflect the real world of work, but I can't.'[14]

In end of life care there is a real risk that the slavish following of guidelines on the treatment of cancer and organ failure could compromise the quality of treatment selection for the individual patient.

2.3 **Assessment of capacity**

Adults are assumed to have capacity until and unless proved otherwise. If doubt has arisen about the patient's capacity for the decision at stake the professional must assess capacity before proceeding further with decision-making. This assessment and subsequent judgement regarding capacity is absolutely crucial because the last stage of decision-making, that of ultimately deciding what investigation or treatment should be provided, follows a different process for patients with and without capacity. Whereas those with capacity will give consent to investigations/treatment finally provided, those lacking capacity will not do so and instead a decision will be made on the basis of their best interests.

It might be argued that capacity should be assessed prior to selection of treatment options, since patients lacking capacity might find some interventions more burdensome, for example due to inability to understand the processes involved or due to disorientation in unfamiliar surroundings. This argument undoubtedly has merit, and so the stages or elements of treatment selection and assessment of capacity will not always occur in the order in which we have described them.

When health care professionals recognize ethical problems in a decision-making situation in end of life care, and are uncertain of how they should act, it often emerges that doubt about the patient's capacity is at least one of the difficulties. If there is any such doubt, the judgement about capacity must be made as soon as the clinical problem has been understood and when treatment options are being considered. The judgement about capacity determines the process by which the final decision will be made—either that for patients with capacity, or that for those lacking capacity.

It is important to understand that capacity is decision-specific, so the assessment is always whether the patient does or does not have capacity for the decision in question. Patients quite often have capacity for simple decisions (such as whether they would like an increase in the dose of the painkiller familiar to them) but not for more complex ones which require consideration of several factors (such as whether to go back into hospital for another attempt at more aggressive diuresis in end-stage heart failure with renal impairment).

Legal tests for capacity may show some slight variation in detail, but they have basic principles in common. We shall describe the test for capacity stipulated by the Mental Capacity Act and therefore used in England and Wales.[15] It is described in the Code of Practice accompanying that Act, Chapter 4.[16] The test is in two stages:

Stage 1: Does the person have an impairment of, or a disturbance in the functioning of, their mind or brain?

A person cannot be judged as lacking capacity unless it can be established that there is such an impairment or disturbance of functioning. This ethically important stipulation protects people who make unusual decisions, or who are eccentric, from being judged as lacking capacity—it acts as a safeguard. End of life care examples of an impairment or disturbance in the functioning of the mind or brain include disorders causing delirium, diminished consciousness, dementia, confusion as an adverse effect of medications, brain tumours, and significant mental illness. Some patients have an impairment such as significant learning disabilities or dementia which pre-dates their terminal illness.

If it is established that the patient does have an impairment or disturbance of functioning of the mind or brain, proceed to:

Stage 2: Does the impairment or disturbance mean that the person is unable to make the specific decision when they need to?

A person is unable to make a decision if they cannot:

1) understand the information relevant to the decision to be made;

2) retain that information in their mind;

3) use or weigh that information as part of the decision-making process; or

4) communicate their decision by any means (including talking, writing, sign language, even blinking).

If the patient is unable to do *any* of these four tasks then he/she lacks capacity for that decision. But prior to that judgement being made, the law stipulates that all practical and appropriate steps must have been taken to help the person make the decision for themselves.[17] Everything practical and appropriate must be done to help the patient to communicate if there is a communication difficulty.[18] So hearing aids, pictorial aids, interpreters, etc., must be supplied and tried! The ethical imperative here is to enable the patient to take the decision if possible.

However, in end of life care there is a difficulty in the stipulation that all practical and appropriate steps must be taken to help patients make the decision themselves. It sometimes happens that metabolic disturbances, such as hypercalcaemia in malignancy, or renal failure, have made the patient unable to do tasks 1–3 because of drowsiness and confusion, and the clinical question is then whether or not to give hospital treatment to try to reverse the metabolic disorder. When a patient is approaching the end of life it may not be clear whether reversal of these disorders is in the interests of a patient whose condition is irreversibly deteriorating and for whom death as a result of the underlying illness is foreseen in the fairly near future. Clinicians faced with the drowsy/confused patient must decide whether or not to give treatment to try to reverse the metabolic abnormality. But the law appears unhelpful here as it instructs that everything 'practical and appropriate' must be done to enable such patients to make their own decision, thus strongly suggesting that the metabolic disturbance causing drowsiness and confusion should be treated—but this is the very decision that the clinicians have identified as at issue. The law in this respect appears to be 'circular'. So clinicians must judge whether it is 'appropriate' to treat the metabolic disturbance, using the patient's best interests as the basis for their decision.

It is important that health care professionals understand that the test for capacity is the same test regardless of the decision to be made. If the decision is more complicated because many factors are relevant, the patient will require greater cognitive and memory powers to have capacity, but the test itself is the same.

A frequent misunderstanding by junior medical staff is the notion that tests of cognitive or memory function, such as the Mini-Mental State Examination, are tests of capacity. They are not and have never been tests of capacity, and it is ethically unacceptable for them to be used as such. Tests of cognitive function or memory are just that—they are not tests for capacity to make a specific decision. An abnormal result in a test of cognitive function may bring decision-making capacity into doubt, so that it will have to be assessed via the proper test. But the result of a test of cognitive function does not prove or disprove capacity. This is obvious when one considers the nature of tasks in tests of cognitive function and memory, for example spelling 'world' backwards, or drawing overlapping pentagons, or subtracting seven serially from 100; ability or inability to perform these tasks cannot, and does not, tell us whether the patient has the crucial abilities required to consider information about a proposed treatment and decide whether to consent to it or refuse it.

Patients' capacity may also fluctuate alongside variations in metabolic abnormalities or alertness, or the effects of medications. It is then important to try to conduct joint decision-making when the patient is most capable of addressing the relevant issues. Such patients can give valid consent when they have capacity, and this can continue to be valid in the short term so that their wishes can be carried out. Similarly, patients with mild to moderate dementia will have capacity if they can understand and retain the information long enough to weigh it up and then communicate their decision. Their consent is likely to be considered morally and legally valid, even though the next day they might not recall the discussion. Obviously, their consent or refusal would be checked again just prior to any treatment or investigation.

Clinicians are all aware that it can be difficult to decide whether or not a patient has capacity for a decision, even though the test is simple and well known.

The judgement about capacity is precisely that—it is a professional judgement. In many cases it is not possible to have certainty. This element of uncertainty is acknowledged and accommodated in law. For example, the Mental Capacity Act Code of Practice stipulates that 'anyone who claims that an individual lacks capacity should be able to provide proof. They need to be able to show *on the balance of probabilities*, that the individual lacks capacity to make a particular decision, at the time it needs to be made (section 2 (4)). This means being able to show that it is more likely than not that the person lacks capacity to make the decision in question.' [italics added][19]

A great deal may rest on the judgement about capacity, especially if a decision is required regarding potentially life-prolonging treatment. Clinicians recognize this and often feel some disquiet that the verdict they reach regarding the patient's capacity is obviously a matter of judgement. They may object that the test for capacity is 'subjective', by which they mean it is a matter of judgement rather than a matter of measuring something like a distance on a scale. But it is part of the role of every health care professional to make this judgement, and to take responsibility for making it. This is particularly apparent in end of life care.

There is sometimes anxiety and uncertainty regarding who should assess capacity and make the judgement. Broadly speaking, the person who should make the assessment is the person who is attempting to make the decision about treatment or care with the patient and who will be carrying out the treatment/care. For example, it frequently falls to nursing staff to decide whether a patient who is apparently refusing medications has capacity to make the decision to take them or not. The nurse will have to judge whether the patient has become confused or paranoid and now lacks capacity, or in fact has capacity and, having reconsidered the issue, has made a decision to refuse the medications. The judgement about capacity is crucial if an agitated and distressed patient is declining to take an anxiolytic (calming) medication. Occupational therapists and physiotherapists working in hospitals may have to judge whether a patient has capacity to choose whether to return home or to go into residential care. The therapists then have to ascertain whether or not the patient has understood the risks of being alone at home for periods, perhaps including the risk of falls, and whether the patient has been able to retain the information and weigh it up. It is the responsibility of all health care professionals involved in end of life care to make the necessary judgements about their patients' capacity when it is in doubt.

We shall now discuss the final stage of decision-making, first for patients who have capacity to make the decision, and then for those who, following assessment, are judged to lack capacity for the decision.

2.4 **Making the final decision with patients who have capacity: consent**

Where the patient has capacity, making the final decision entails and requires the obtaining of the patient's consent for the treatment chosen from the options offered. What is meant by 'consent'? We touched on this issue in Section 1.4.i) but will now examine it in more detail.

The sense of consent to be found in ordinary speech is 'agreeing to' or 'accepting'. If you say to your colleague: 'Shall we go for coffee now?' and your colleague says 'OK', your colleague has consented as far as ordinary language goes. The point is that in ordinary speech consent does not entail *rights*. In medicine this sense might be illustrated by contexts in which the doctor says 'I am proposing to do X and Y' or 'I have just done X and Y. Is that OK?', and the patient weakly says 'Yes, thank you doctor' without really considering, or perhaps feeling able to consider, what is proposed. This would not now be regarded as a valid consent in current medical practice.

There is a second way of looking at consent, now regarded as central and essential to the medical context. It is applicable whenever the patient has capacity. This is a partnership model[20] and it is effectively 'consent as shared decision-making.' It has two elements:

1 The doctor identifies investigations and treatment options likely to result in overall benefit to the patient, having listened to the patient's concerns and views. The doctor then sets out, for each option, the potential benefits, harms and risks and may recommend a particular option. The patient weighs up this information alongside personal preferences and priorities. Discussion is needed to provide clarification for both parties and to consider any further options or compromise solutions. This type of discussion is necessary but not sufficient for partnership (shared) decision-making.

2 The second necessary condition is that this discussion results in the activating of a socially or often a legally sanctioned procedure. We can call this procedure the giving or the refusing of *permission*. These two conditions are together necessary and sufficient for this sense of consent. We should like to note some points about it.

(a) Permission is given by both patient and doctor. The doctor permits treatment to be provided via the service, and the patient gives permission for it to be administered to his own body. Each may permit treatment or not.

(b) Permission is a *normative* term. This means that it acts to direct human conduct and derives from an underlying basis of rules, rights and duties. It is not like 'agreeing' or 'accepting' which are non-normative. I can accept a drink or agree to go to the cinema without any question of *rights*. But to give permission is to confer a right. Thus the patient gives or refuses the doctor a right to intervene (i.e. to carry out an investigation or treatment), and the doctor gives the patient the right to have the investigation/treatment(s) offered.

(c) The norms (moral rules) in question must be socially and, in the end, legally sanctioned or legitimized by public policy. In other words, not only must the parties know and agree about the procedures or treatments offered, *society* more generally must know and agree to the general ethical framework for the practice of consenting to, or refusing, treatment.

We have identified the patient's giving of permission as a necessary element of the process of 'consent as shared decision-making'. But it should not be taken in isolation from the discussion element. The GMC makes this point clear in the following paragraph in its guidance on consent:[21]

> You must work in partnership with your patients. You should discuss with them their condition and treatment options in a way they can understand, and respect their right to make decisions about their care. You should see getting their consent as an important part of the process of discussion and decision-making, rather than as something that happens in isolation.

This point is particularly important in end of life care, where the process of discussion is essential to establish which treatment or care options will further one or more of the three aims of health care and will also most accord with the patient's priorities, values and preferences.

Consent as shared decision-making seems the most satisfactory model for consent in the end of life care context where the patient has capacity. There are, however, four difficulties with this solution, concerning: the amount of information the patient should be given (Section 2.4.i); patients who continue to request treatment that is clinically inappropriate (Section 2.4.ii); the question of whether patients have not just a right to give consent but a duty to do so (Section 2.4.iii); patients who lack capacity to consent. We shall discuss the last difficulty in Section 2.5.

2.4.i How much information?

There are particular problems with disclosure of information in end of life care; patients may not want some of the information, perhaps as a result of anxiety, fear or general distress, or they may be exhausted and so find concentrating on information burdensome, even for short periods. Professionals will seek guidance on the following: the nature of information which must be disclosed in order for consent to be ethically (and legally) valid; what it is good practice to disclose (but where there is some discretion); what should be done where patients decline information; possible justifications for proceeding with treatment with the patient's agreement but without disclosure of crucial information.

In the UK, the GMC guidance on consent serves as the professional standard for disclosure; unfortunately its meaning is not adequately clear because it does not explain the meaning of crucial terms used.

The current guidance states that:

> You *must* give patients the information they *want* or *need* about: the diagnosis and prognosis . . . options for treating or managing the condition, including the option not to treat . . . the potential benefits, risks and burdens, and the likelihood of success, for each option. [italics added][22]

The guidance stipulates that 'must' indicates an 'overriding' duty or principle. The term 'overriding' here implies that the obligation overrides other moral considerations and principles, presumably including whether the patient wants the information or could be harmed by it.

So the guidance is stating that there is an obligation, which overrides other obligations, to disclose information which the patient 'wants' or 'needs'. The instruction that patients must be given information that they want is not ethically contentious or complex. By contrast, the term 'need' is highly problematic because the GMC does not give any criteria by which a doctor could judge whether a patient 'needs' an item of information for a particular decision. For example, is the standard for 'need' that which a reasonable person would consider necessary to make the decision, or is it particular to the individual patient and linked to what is wanted, or is it some sort of legal standard? The term implies that without the information which is 'needed' the patient's consent is not valid. Paragraph 9 lists many items of information which doctors 'must' give to patients if they 'want or need' it, but this fails to resolve uncertainty as doctors are not told how to determine whether an item of information is 'needed' or 'necessary' for valid decision-making.

The seriousness of this uncertainty is illustrated by a later instruction in paragraph 44:

> Before accepting a patient's consent, you must consider whether they have been given the information they want or need, and how well they understand the details and implications of what is proposed.

The ethical difficulty here is that unless the doctor accepts the patient's consent (having judged it to be valid), the patient cannot receive the treatment, since for patients with capacity giving consent is effectively a condition of receiving treatment. The 'must' means that doctors have an overriding duty to satisfy themselves that patients have received and understood the information they wanted or needed as a condition of judging that consent is valid. Unless they are thus satisfied, doctors cannot proceed with the intervention. But the doctors do not know how to judge what information is 'needed', so may feel frustrated that they are not equipped to judge whether consent can be deemed valid or not. Comment has been made that in the GMC guidance details are sparse and the advice is non-specific, with no detail about the suggested risk thresholds for specifying the probability of harm.[23] We would also stress that lack of criteria by which to determine what information is 'needed' greatly reduces the usefulness of this guidance for clinical practice and as a standard by which doctors will be judged.

There is some clarity regarding information which 'must' be disclosed, meaning that there is an 'overriding duty' to disclose it. Paragraph 32 states: 'You must tell patients if an investigation or treatment might result in a serious adverse outcome, even if the likelihood is very small'.[24] A serious adverse outcome is described in a note as 'an adverse outcome resulting in death, permanent or long-term physical disability or disfigurement, medium- or long-term pain, or admission to hospital; or other outcomes with long-term or permanent effect on a patient's employment, social or personal life.'[25] In addition, paragraph 29 lists as adverse outcomes which 'must' be disclosed: side-effects and complications of the treatment, and the risk of failure of the intervention to achieve the desired aim. However, the range of 'seriousness' is quite large. For example, a patient might require hospital admission because of a life-threatening condition, such as neutropenic sepsis following chemotherapy, or because of a much less serious (but nevertheless distressing) problem such as severe constipation secondary to opiates—both would count as 'serious' adverse outcomes which 'must' be disclosed.

With regard to outcomes not falling into the category of 'serious', paragraph 32 advises that 'You should also tell patients about less serious side effects or complications if they occur frequently, and explain what the patient should do if they experience any of them'. 'You should', according to the guidance, indicates either how doctors will meet the overriding duty to disclose information, *or* that the duty or principle will not apply in all circumstances, and it also covers situations where factors outside the doctor's control may affect whether it is possible to comply with the guidance. The problem is that these two meanings are quite different—readers cannot know which meaning is intended here, or elsewhere in the guidance.[26]

In contrast to the GMC professional standard for disclosure, guidance on communication skills instructs that 'professionals need to identify those who wish to take part in decisions and respect those who wish the clinician to take decisions for them.' In advising on effective interview techniques it advises 'that giving information during an interview reduces the likelihood of further disclosure'[27] of the patient's feelings. Thus guidance on communication skills actually discourages disclosure of information about treatment, especially where patients do not want much involvement/information in decision-making. Professionals may be forgiven for feeling confused!

GMC guidance on the situation where patients decline information (paragraphs 13–17) does not resolve the issue. It explains that doctors should try to find out why information is being declined and should explain to patients why it is important that it be disclosed. It then advises that where patients still do not want to know in detail about their condition or the treatment, 'you should respect their wishes, as far as possible. But you *must* still give them the information they *need* in order to give their consent to a proposed investigation or treatment.' (italics added). The 'must' here implies an overriding duty to disclose to patients the information that they 'need', even if they do not want disclosure. However, the guidance then goes on to advise that where patients decline information they must be informed that their consent may not be valid, and that doctors must justify and record why information was withheld. It recommends that doctors consider whether patients could be given the information later, 'without causing them serious harm', implying that serious harm could be a justification for non-disclosure. But if there are justifications for non-disclosure, then the 'must' to disclose cannot, logically, be an *overriding* duty.

The GMC guidance does make it clear that information should not be withheld because relatives, partners, friends or carers of the patient request that it be withheld.[28] This last instruction is ethically essential in end of life care, where well-meaning family members may try to prevent patients being given information about prognosis and the limited potential of treatment to alter the course of the illness.

We had hoped in Part 1 of this book to discuss consensus professional guidance and its ethical implications in end of life care. However, we remain unclear as to how GMC guidance on this issue should be interpreted and enacted, and we note that guidance on communication skills runs contrary to GMC standards for disclosure. We conclude that there is currently no real professional consensus on this issue.

Lack of consensus (and clear guidance) may be contributing to failure to disclose information which would reasonably be required for adequately informed consent. For example, it is important when considering treatment options that patients are given a realistic understanding of the overall prognosis of their illness. There is evidence of lack of disclosure of prognosis in oncology (see Section 4.4.i). Similar problems seem to occur in primary care; identified barriers to disclosure include concerns about causing distress and damaging hope, prognostic uncertainty in chronic illness, plus lack of time for the discussions.[29] Even though a chronic illness may be expected to cause death, prognostic uncertainty regarding time scales does appear to discourage professionals from disclosing the true prognosis, for example in heart failure.[30] This is ethically important.

It is reasonable to ask if withholding information about a terminal prognosis could ever be morally justified. Daniel Sokol, a lecturer in medical ethics and law, attempted to devise guidance on deception regarding 'grim truths', and even produced an algorithm summarizing it.[31] He used the term 'non-lying deception' which would encompass such intentional withholding of crucial information. His list of justifications for deception (which are proposed, but which will only rarely justify the deception when everything is considered) include preventing great physical or psychological harm to the patient, reducing anxiety and great stress, and preserving or enhancing hope. The moral problem with all of these is that ill-informed patients are not equipped to make decisions which accord with their own values if they do not realize that their current illness is likely to result in death in the foreseeable future. So deception remains extremely difficult to justify when decisions are at stake. We return to the issue of disclosure of prognostic information in the context of potentially life-prolonging treatment in Section 4.4.i.

Considering now the disclosure of information about adverse outcomes, there is some evidence of ethically important non-disclosure regarding palliative chemotherapy. For example, the high risks of death and toxicity resulting from chemotherapy given to very sick patients were identified in the 2008 UK National Confidential Enquiry into Patient Outcome and Death (NCEPOD) analysis of data from 600 patients who died within 30 days of receiving chemotherapy. The expert panel considered that chemotherapy had probably caused or hastened death in 27% of the patients studied, most of whom were receiving it as palliative rather than curative treatment. In addition, 43% of patients had substantial toxicity in relation to treatment. With regard to the role of patients in decision-making, the report emphasizes that 'there is a concern that they might not have had sufficient information to allow them to balance the burdens and benefits of treatment.'[32] This example illustrates why it is ethically so important that patients are informed of potentially serious adverse outcomes, and of the likelihood that the treatment will not achieve its aim.

The moral basis for an obligation to provide this information is the fact that patients cannot judge what they do and do not want done to themselves without some crucial information about benefits, harms, and risks. Serious adverse outcomes are of such major significance for patients that it can be argued that they must be given information about them in order to be able to make a decision. In end of life care it is particularly important that patients give (or withhold) consent in a 'morally valid' sense for two reasons.

The first is that patients with incurable and life-threatening illness may be offered burdensome and risky treatments which have some prospect of prolonging life, but where the chance of response to the treatment is low (e.g. 30% or less). Palliative chemotherapy regimes are an obvious example. In this situation the likelihood of harm and risk actually exceeds the likelihood of benefit, so there is a very strong moral argument in support of an obligation to give patients information about the high probability that the intervention will fail to achieve the desired aim, as well as serious adverse outcomes and other significant adverse effects.

The second reason is that in end of life care 'time is running out'. If patients do not benefit from treatments, and particularly if adverse outcomes or burdens ensue, then life which they could have had in greater comfort and/or independence has been irrevocably lost. It cannot be regained. The loss of the last potential 'good living time' is rightly seen as a major loss.

Although these are excellent reasons to support disclosure, we have noted the contrary ideas portrayed in 'communication skills' teaching, and the reasonable points that patients might genuinely be so exhausted that considering other than minimal information is burdensome, or they may be very anxious and declining disclosure as it entails 'bad news'. These are the sort of situations which the BMA is probably trying to accommodate in its guidance on decisions pertaining to withholding and withdrawing life-prolonging treatment. It states that patients should be encouraged to be involved in decision-making to the extent to which they feel comfortable.[33] This implies that where patients do not feel comfortable with such involvement, then they do not have to be involved, with the implication that information need not be given. Authors from the background of clinical ethics have proposed that although patients are fully entitled to take an active role in decision-making about treatment, they are not required to do so.[34] Even the GMC guidance states that 'How much information you share with patients will vary, depending on their individual circumstances.'[35] So there are good arguments for giving professionals some discretion, but how much discretion should be granted?

There is clearly a need for some discretion, based on clinical judgement, about what patients ought to be told. Sokol has commented that overreliance on law and professional guidelines tends to stifle moral deliberation and reflection, which are essential to good clinical practice.[36] In the end, professionals must decide what information should be disclosed, including when patients are severely exhausted or refusing information. Communicating risk to patients can also be difficult; helpful guidance stresses the importance of honesty and of exploring the patient's understanding of, and reaction to, the information.[37] It is obvious that consent can never be 'fully' informed as it would be impractical and burdensome to try to convey all information. Readers wishing to reflect on these issues might wish to read a helpful paper by Baroness O'Neill on the limits of informed consent.[38]

In the past, doctors were permitted a large measure of discretion with regard to disclosure. But current GMC guidance now implies that if patients are not given information which they 'need' or which they 'must' be given in order for consent to be valid, then the intervention cannot proceed. Thus it appears that an early twentieth century model of 'benevolent paternalism' may not now ever be acceptable, even in the end of life situation. In a 'benevolent paternalism' model, doctors offered a treatment plan based on their judgement of what was the best option for that patient, they judged how much information to disclose, and they were free to withhold information that the patient did not want. The patient either agreed to the treatment plan or (uncommonly) refused it. In the twenty-first century this model appears to have been rejected, even in those circumstances where it might best serve the interests of exhausted patients in need of symptom control; the right to give informed consent has arguably moved too far towards a duty to do so as a prerequisite of receiving treatment. (See also Sections 2.4.iii below, and 4.4.i and 5.2 on disclosure of information pertinent to life-prolonging treatment and symptom control respectively.)

We have said much about 'what' information ought to be communicated, but nothing so far about the ethically important issue of 'how' it ought to be communicated. It is obvious that information should be given sensitively and with compassion. But much has been said and written in recent years about 'communication skills', and the impression is sometimes given that such skills can and should be acquired from courses. So there are 'communication skills courses' and even 'advanced communication skills' courses, although evaluations indicate limited transfer of the acquired 'skills' back into the workplace.[39] Certainly there are basic skills which can be acquired from such courses, but there is an ethical argument that professionals should still communicate genuinely, rather than being taught a pattern of verbal and non-verbal behaviours designed to make the patient believe that the professional is 'caring'. Furthermore, patients are likely to be aware of being addressed by a professional who is genuinely compassionate and sensitive, as opposed to a professional who has simply learned a pattern of behaviour designed to give that impression.

It is possible that the focus on 'what' information must or should be given will eclipse the ethically important factor of 'how' it is imparted. The fact that we have mentioned this issue last in this section should not be taken to imply that 'how' the professional imparts information is ethically less significant than what is imparted.

2.4.ii The continuing request for what is clinically inappropriate

This second difficulty will arise if the patient or relatives persist in requesting a certain treatment which the doctor thinks is not clinically appropriate. Public health experts have acknowledged that patients' preferences do not exactly overlap with good quality care, and that some of their wishes would be detrimental to them if doctors were to comply. In other words, what patients say they want is sometimes not the same as good quality care.[40] There cannot in this situation be shared decision-making in the sense that the doctor cannot agree to the patient's request, so must decline 'permission' for himself and the service to provide the treatment. The doctor cannot 'share' responsibility for giving a treatment which is not clinically appropriate. This situation creates a challenge to the doctor's ability to communicate with the patient and relatives. The GMC suggests the following reasonable approach:

> If the patient asks for a treatment that the doctor considers would not be of overall benefit to them, the doctor should discuss the issues with the patient and explore the reasons for their request. If, after discussion, the doctor still considers that the treatment would not be of overall benefit to the patient, they do not have to provide the treatment. But they should explain their reasons to the patient, and explain any other options that are available, including the option to seek a second opinion.[41]

The vast majority of patients will in the end accept doctors' advice. In the rare situations in which doctors' advice is not accepted and patients persists in the request, then doctors must hold firmly to their considered professional judgement; doctors will then be supported in the courts, at least in the UK.[42] We have already noted, in relation to decisions regarding life-prolonging treatment, that doctors ought to offer and provide only those treatments where the possible benefits outweigh the harms or risks, and that doctors should avoid provision of treatments where there is no foreseen net benefit to the patient.[43] It can be argued that rather than *not having* an obligation to provide treatment which is clinically inappropriate, the doctor instead *has* an obligation not to provide such treatment. The basis of this obligation is, of course, the obligation not to cause net harm to patients. Authors writing on medical ethics have thus stated 'there will be some occasions in which acquiescence to a requested intervention against one's clinical or ethical judgement will be abrogation of one's duty as a doctor.'[44] We return to this issue in Section 4.4.ii.

2.4.iii **A right to consent or a duty to do so?**

The third difficulty concerns a possible shift from the idea that a patient has a right to give adequately informed consent to the idea that the patient has a duty to do so. In the latter case the giving of informed consent becomes a precondition of receiving any treatment. We can understand why this view has gained ground: it protects the doctor from the threats of litigation and criticism; it ensures that patients really do know what they are giving permission for; and it seems an inevitable outcome of regulations designed to ensure that patients are given adequate information.

But in health care generally, and especially in end of life care, the notion of duty to consent as a precondition of receiving treatment is arguably an undesirable outcome of ruling that the patient must have adequate information. As we have already noted, consent would probably be judged invalid if information about serious adverse outcomes were withheld; this leads directly to the consequence that patients must receive such information as a precondition of treatment. Seen in this light, it does appear that the right to give consent to treatment is well on the way to transforming into a duty to give consent as a precondition of treatment. It has been argued by bioethicists that the attempt to remove 'medical paternalism' in decision-making is in danger of replacing it with an equally (or possibly even more) unacceptable paternalism![45]

The fourth difficulty we noted (at the end of Section 2.4) with decision-making through the consent process is that it cannot function where patients lack capacity to make their own choices. In end of life care, many patients will at some time lack capacity to consent to or refuse treatment and care options. Furthermore, clinical situations recognized as ethically complex often pertain to decisions made on behalf of patients who lack capacity. This area requires a section on its own.

2.5 **Making the final decision: patients without capacity**

People of different cultures approach decision-making for patients who lack capacity in slightly different ways, so that socially sanctioned professional conduct in this matter does differ in detail between countries. This is reflected in differences in law. Differences in culture and law are perhaps most obvious in the context of end of life care. But in order to be truly effective, any law governing decision-making for adults who lack capacity must be comprehensive. It must govern the following issues:

- the basis for the judgement of capacity, or lack of it, for the decision in question and the process of making that judgement;

- the identity of the person responsible for making the judgement about capacity;
- who takes responsibility for making health care decisions for the adult patient who lacks capacity (e.g. nearest relative, or health care professional);
- the basis on which the decision must be taken (e.g. on the basis of what is in the patient's best interests, or on the basis of what the patient would have chosen; the latter is sometimes called a 'substitute judgement');
- what provision there should be for a person who still has capacity to appoint someone to consent to or refuse treatment on behalf of that person if the latter should lose capacity in the future;
- what provision there should be for persons who have capacity to influence decision-making at a future time when they lack capacity, by means of verbal or written advance statements including advance decisions to refuse specific treatments;
- what recourse there should be to a court of law to resolve disputes or enduring uncertainty regarding either the judgement of capacity or a particular decision for a patient who lacks capacity.

Readers will need to be aware of the law and professional guidance of their own country in respect of these various issues. We shall describe some features of the Mental Capacity Act 2005 (which is the UK law for England and Wales, but not for Scotland) which are of particular interest and relevance for ethics in end of life care.[46] We will not attempt a comprehensive review of the Act, since to do so would not be relevant to some readers and our purpose is not to review health care law. But we will use this recent Act as an example of how the issues listed above may be addressed. Since we have already discussed the judgement of capacity, we will proceed now to the question of who makes the decision.

Under the Act the person who takes responsibility for the decision for the patient who lacks capacity is normally the health care professional responsible for carrying out the particular treatment or procedure. This does seem the most ethically appropriate solution. So if a urologist is caring for a patient who lacks capacity because of renal failure due to urinary tract obstruction by pelvic malignancy, the person who is the decision-maker regarding the insertion of nephrostomies or ureteric stents is actually the person who conducts the procedure. This person might be a radiologist. If a patient is close to death and various medications have been prescribed to be given as needed to alleviate distress, then the decision-maker at administration of each medication is actually the nurse who will choose and give it from the range of drugs prescribed.

There are three exceptions to this general rule conferring decision-making responsibility on the health care professional. At the time of writing they are not commonly encountered in end of life care. The first exception is where the patient has appointed someone as Lasting Power of Attorney with authority to make the health care decision in question; that attorney will consent to or refuse the treatment on behalf of the patient. In this situation the attorney decides in lieu of the patient and so consents to or refuses treatment on behalf of the patient. In a sense, the decision-making method more closely resembles that for patients with capacity, but attornies must base their decision on the best interests of the patient. The second exception is where the Court of Protection has become involved and has appointed a deputy to make decisions, which must also be based on the patient's best interests. The third exception is where the patient has made a legally binding advance refusal of the particular treatment in question and that refusal is valid and applicable in the circumstances. In this last case the patient has effectively made the decision in advance by refusing the specific treatment in the circumstances which have arisen. Laws in other countries will cover these same issues, but will differ in details.

The moral and legal responsibility for the decision will be carried by one individual, not by 'the team', even though the views of members of the health care team will be taken into account. We discuss the issue of teams and decision-making further in Section 4.1.

With regard to the basis of the decision (fourth issue on our list), the Act stipulates that where the patient lacks capacity the basis for the decision must be the 'best interests' of the patient. The basis is not 'what the patient would have chosen', sometimes called a 'substitute judgement',[47] although laws of some other jurisdictions use this alternative basis. The substitute judgement is difficult to make—it is very frequently uncertain what decision the patient would have made. Moreover, occasionally the decision which it is thought the patient would have made does not accord with the patient's best interests. This situation can happen because we all sometimes make decisions which are not in our best interests. For example, we might make an unwise decision because of overwhelming desires, or we might make a very altruistic decision which benefits others but entails some harm to ourselves. In its favour, the 'substitute judgement' basis ensures that the decision most closely reflects what the patient would have decided, including an unwise or altruistic decision, so it is not paternalistic. The 'best interests' basis is open to the charge of paternalism; the difficulty of determining what is in the patient's best interests remains; and it can be excessively individualistic as the decision must be based only on the interests of the patient, to the exclusion of the interests of others.

In making the best interests judgement, the health care professional must take into account all the relevant circumstances (including the benefits, harms and risks of the treatment options in the selected range) plus whatever can be known of the patient's wishes, feelings, beliefs and values. In determining the latter it is necessary to consult (if practical and appropriate) close relatives and friends of the patient and those engaged in caring for the patient. If a patient has no close friends or family whom it is appropriate to consult, then if a serious medical treatment decision is at stake or if a specific sort of decision regarding location of care is required, an Independent Mental Capacity Advocate must be appointed. This advocate is not a decision-maker, but represents that patient who would otherwise be in a highly vulnerable position. In best interests judgements, professionals must also take into account any verbal or written advance statement the patient made previously.

There is, of course, a responsibility to respect the confidentiality of the patient even though the latter has lost capacity. But consulting close family and friends about the patient's wishes, feelings, beliefs and values, and overall best interests in the current situation necessarily involves divulging much information to those friends and relatives. An ethically important conflict of duties may arise. The Act does not indicate how this should be resolved; its Code of Practice merely reminds professionals that 'it would not be right to share every piece of information with everyone'.[48] An ethically reasonable compromise would appear to be disclosure of that which friends and family 'need to know' so as to inform the best interests decision, unless the professional has reason to believe that the patient would not have wished disclosure to certain parties. This is the position the BMA takes in its guidance on decision-making about life-prolonging treatment, which stipulates that where there is evidence that the patient did not want information shared this 'must' be respected. The BMA notes that when information is 'sensitive' a professional judgement must be made about 'how much information the patient is likely to want passed on to whom.'[49] Guidance on good practice regarding confidentiality concurs with the view that information which patients do not want disclosed to their family should not be disclosed.[50] Patients requesting non-disclosure to certain individuals may not wish those persons to be involved in decision-making, and it may be helpful to clarify this issue prior to loss of capacity.

In the context of end of life care, some of the most difficult decisions for patients who lack capacity arise in relation to treatments which have the potential to sustain or prolong life for a period. We discuss these in Section 4.5, but note here that the Act stipulates that professionals making decisions about life-sustaining treatment must not be motivated by a desire to bring about the person's death for whatever reason. So motivation to bring about the patient's death is unlawful even if the root of such motivation is compassion. This is an example of a legal prohibition of euthanasia for patients who lack capacity.

A further stipulation in relation to life-sustaining treatment is that decision-makers 'should not make assumptions about the patient's quality of life.'[51] This is challenging to those health care professionals who consider that the notion of 'quality of life' is useful in making such decisions. The stipulation appears in the Act's Code of Practice and so has legal force. It is of considerable ethical importance so we shall discuss it in more detail in the context of decisions regarding life-prolonging treatment in Section 4.5.i.

Another ethically significant feature of the Act, and one which is challenging to professionals who believe that they must also promote the welfare of the patient's family, is that this law explicitly requires that the decision must be based only on the patient's best interests, not on the interests of others such as relatives. Where there is clear evidence that the patient would have considered the interests of the relatives to be important, this would be taken into account, as explained in the Code of Practice.[52] So it is very difficult, under this Act, to make a decision which is neutral (or slightly harmful) where the patient is concerned but which would clearly be of great benefit to the relatives. This law is designed to protect the interests of the patient who lacks capacity against the pursuit of the interests of any other parties, including relatives, other patients, the health care professionals concerned and the community in general.

The ethical significance of the Act's protection of the patient's interests is the cost in terms of adverse effects on the welfare/interests of all other parties. The Act's stipulation is in contrast to ordinary morality, where we normally judge that we should give consideration to the interests of all parties in a morally difficult situation. We do not normally assume or believe that the interests of a single person should necessarily override the interests of others. Any law which gives exclusive protection to the interests of the patient lacking capacity necessarily sacrifices the interests of other parties, including other patients to whom professionals owe an equal duty of care. This is ethically important in relation to care for relatives and in relation to resource distribution. We shall mention it again in those contexts (Sections 8.2.v, 8.2.vi, and 10.3).

Turning to the fifth and sixth issues, which any law relating to patients who lack capacity must govern, we have already explained that: the Act enables the patient to appoint someone to act as an attorney to consent to or refuse treatment on the patient's behalf; decision-makers must take advance statements into account; advance decisions to refuse specific treatment are legally binding on professionals provided they meet the Act's requirements regarding formulation, validity and applicability (see Chapter 7).

Normally the decision-makers' judgement about what is in the patient's best interests determines what is done. But if decision-making proves extremely difficult, or if there is unresolved conflict between either health care professionals themselves, or between professionals and relatives of the patient, an application can be made to a special court (called the Court of Protection), to make the final decision.

2.6 Conclusions

1) The moral quality of a clinical decision is dependent on the process of that decision and not only on the outcome. We are accountable and responsible for the way in which our decisions are reached.

2) In end of life care, outcomes are multifactorial and unpredictable. Professionals are accountable for the outcome only to the extent that their decision did, of itself, influence the outcome.

3) Our understanding of the patient's experience will always be limited, but sensitive communication and acceptance of the patient's views and priorities are essential. Taking account of the patient's views, the professional uses knowledge, experience and clinical judgement to identify which treatment options are likely to result in overall benefit.

4) The doctor explains the options to the patient with capacity, setting out the potential benefits, harms and risks of each option. The patient weighs up the information and decides whether to consent to any option. Where the patient lacks capacity, decisions are made in the patient's best interests.

5) Treatment cannot be imposed on the patient with capacity who refuses it. Equally, professionals cannot be forced to give treatment which they conscientiously judge is contrary to the patient's best interests, the latter being based on a benefits to harms/risks calculus.

References

1. Stirrat GM, Gill R (2005). Autonomy in medical ethics after O'Neill. *J Med Ethics* **31**:127–130.
2. General Medical Council (2008). *Consent: patients and doctors making decisions together.* General Medical Council, London para. 5a.
3. Spiegel D, Harrington A (2008). What is the placebo worth? *BMJ* **336**:967–8.
4. Elwyn G, Buetow S, Hibbard J, Wensing M (2007). Respecting the subjective: quality measurement from the patient's perspective. *BMJ* **335**:1021–2.
5. GMC, op. cit. (ref. 2), para. 5b.
6. General Medical Council (2002). *Withholding and withdrawing life-prolonging treatments.* GMC, London, para. 9.

7. GMC, op. cit. (ref. 2), para. 8b.

8. GMC, op. cit. (ref. 2), para. 31.

9. Stirrat, Gill, op. cit. (ref. 1), p. 129.

10. Sokol D (2008). Clarifying best interests. *BMJ* **337**:a994.

11. Coulter A, Ellins J (2007). Effectiveness of strategies for informing, educating, and involving patients. *BMJ* **335**:24–7.

12. Bate P, Robert G (2005). Choice: more can mean less. *BMJ* **331**:1488–9.

13. Sokol D (2008). Clarifying best interests. *BMJ* **337**:a994.

14. Spence D (2008). Medicine's living death. *BMJ* **337**:a674.

15. UK Government (2005). Mental Capacity Act. Office of Public Sector Information, London.

16. Department for Constitutional Affairs (2007). Mental Capacity Act 2005 Code of Practice. The Stationery Office, Norwich.

17. DCA, op. cit. (ref. 16), para. 3.8.

18. DCA, op. cit. (ref. 16), para. 4.13.

19. DCA, op. cit. (ref. 16), para. 4.10.

20. GMC, op. cit. (ref. 2), para. 3–5.

21. GMC, op. cit. (ref. 2), p. 5.

22. GMC, op. cit. (ref. 2), para. 9.

23. Elwyn G (2008). Patient consent—decision or assumption? *BMJ* **336**:1260.

24. GMC, op. cit. (ref. 2), para. 32.

25. GMC, op. cit. (ref. 2), endnote 9.

26. GMC, op. cit. (ref. 2), p. 5.

27. Heaven C, Maguire P (2008). Communication issues. In Lloyd-Williams M (ed.), *Psychosocial issues in palliative care.* Oxford University Press, Oxford, pp. 23, 32.

28. GMC, op. cit. (ref. 2), para. 16.

29. Murray SA, Boyd K, Sheikh A (2005). Palliative care in chronic illness. *BMJ* **330**:622–2.

30. Zambroski CH (2006). Managing beyond an uncertain illness trajectory: palliative care in advanced heart failure. *International Journal of Palliative Nursing* **12**:566–572.

31. Sokol D (2007). Can deceiving patients be morally acceptable? *BMJ* **334**:984–6.

32. National Confidential Enquiry into Patient Outcome and Death (2008). *For better, for worse?* NCEPOD, London, p. 8.

33. British Medical Association (2007). *Withdrawing and withholding life-prolonging medical treatment,* 3rd edn. Blackwell, Oxford, pp. 31–2.

34. Stirrat G, Gill R (2005). op. cit. p. 128.

35. GMC, op. cit. (ref. 2), para. 7.

36. Sokol D (2008). What does the law say? *BMJ* **337**:a617.

37. Thomson R, Edwards A, Grey J (2005). Risk communication in the clinical consultation. *Clin Med* **5**:465–9.

38. O'Neill O (2003). Some limits of informed consent. *J Med Ethics* **29**:4–7.

39. Heaven, Maguire, op. cit. (ref. 27), pp. 37–41.

40. Elwyn *et al.,* op. cit. (ref. 4), p. 1021.

41. GMC, op. cit. (ref. 2), para. 5 d.

42. Mr Leslie Burke v GMC [2005] EWCA Civ 1003.

43. GMC, op. cit. (ref. 6), para. 9.

44. Stirrat, Gill, op. cit. (ref. 1), p. 130.

45. Stirrat, Gill, op. cit. (ref. 1), p. 128.

46. UK Government, op. cit. (ref. 15).

47. Beauchamp TL, Childress JF (2009). *Principles of biomedical ethics*, 6th edn. Oxford University Press, Oxford, pp. 136–8.

48. DCA, op. cit. (ref. 16), p. 66.

49. BMA, op. cit. (ref. 33), p. 33.

50. Bourke J, Wessely S (2008). Confidentiality. *BMJ* **336**:888–91.

51. DCA, op. cit. (ref. 16), p. 65.

52. DCA, op. cit. (ref. 16), p. 83.

Three logical distinctions in decision-making

There are three logical distinctions with ethical significance which are of considerable importance in decision-making in end of life care, and about which a consensus has evolved. They are the distinctions between intending and foreseeing a consequence, between acts and omissions, and between killing and letting die. An understanding of these distinctions is essential for clinical practice in end of life care; it is also necessary for the ethical justification of day-to-day decisions in this context. We shall now outline these distinctions.

3.1 Intended and foreseen consequences: doctrine of double effect

At the outset of this discussion we note again the three central aims of health care, namely the relief of suffering, prolongation of life and maintenance or restoration of function. Professionals intend to bring about one or more of these aims/benefits. We have stressed that treatment/care options should be offered on the basis of the likely positive balance of benefit compared with the harms and risks associated with the treatment for the particular patient in the clinical circumstances. Whereas professionals intend the overall benefit which is their aim, they foresee but do not intend the harms and risks entailed in the treatment/care. Since we are accountable for our part in decision-making and in providing treatment, foreseen harms and risks entailed in the investigation/ treatment proposed must be justified by the intended relative benefit. This is so with virtually all medical and nursing interventions.

It is helpful to consider general health care examples to illustrate the important and well-understood difference between intending and foreseeing an outcome. Antibiotics are often prescribed to combat infection, with the intentions of prolonging life and alleviating suffering. But in some cases they may be associated with harms such as gastrointestinal upset, risks of allergy, or infection by organisms such as *Clostridium difficile*. It is understood that the doctor intends only the benefits. No reasonable person would suggest that the doctor 'intends' that the patient should suffer gastrointestinal side-effects, develop an allergic reaction or suffer *C. difficile*-associated diarrhoea. The harms and risks are foreseen but definitely not intended. Similarly, surgeons and anaesthetists intend the benefits of operations, whereas they foresee, but do not intend, the inevitable harms and risks of the surgery and the anaesthetic. The distinction between intending and foreseeing is still clear even when the harms and risks are inevitable and inescapable (although of course attempts will be made to ameliorate or minimize them). The different concepts of intending and foreseeing are well understood in ordinary language and in health care.

In end of life care, treatment given with the intention of prolonging life or alleviating suffering can be associated with the risk that life may be shortened by adverse effects of treatment. For example, in the study of the deaths within 30 days of chemotherapy, already mentioned in Section 2.4.i, it was found that death was hastened or caused by the chemotherapy in 27% of cases. Although this proportion is worryingly high, no-one would suggest that the oncologists intended that the patients should die sooner because of the treatment, even though they would have foreseen the harms (toxicity) and risks (especially neutropenic sepsis) associated with the treatment.

Medications given to alleviate suffering are generally associated with lesser risks of shortening life than risky but potentially life-prolonging treatments. However, it may rarely occur that sedation given to alleviate mental anguish or agitated delirium, or sedation plus high-dose opiate analgesia for pain unrelieved by all other means, could shorten life by reducing fluid intake, increasing the likelihood of hypostatic pneumonia and perhaps by respiratory depression. Regarding opiate analgesia, sedation may result as an adverse effect; respiratory depression due specifically to opiates would be very rare with proper use. Sometimes sedation given to alleviate distress due to respiratory failure could shorten life by causing respiratory depression, for example where there is tracheal obstruction by tumour, or when the patient has respiratory failure due to chronic obstructive pulmonary disease which is refractory to treatment.

Near the end of life, some particularly unpleasant symptoms might also require medications that cause sedation as a side-effect. For example, intractable fitting due to advanced cerebral tumours can occur. Sometimes it is best controlled (or only controlled) by continuous subcutaneous infusion of benzodiazepines such as midazolam, which is then likely to cause sedation which in turn could shorten life (albeit by only a little).

It is clear that intentional overdoses either of sedatives or of analgesics are not morally justified. Proper practice is the use of analgesics for pain relief, and sedatives for agitation/delirium, or emotional anguish; analgesics should not be used in doses in excess of those needed for pain relief in order to achieve a sedative effect. Distress due to catastrophic events such as tracheal obstruction and haemorrhage may be treated with both morphine and sedation. Much has been learned about the relief of intractable symptoms by the skilled use of medications and careful dose titration. Where symptom control is proving complex or difficult, advice should be sought from specialist palliative medicine physicians, who are available for such consultation in the UK.

In the examples where medications to alleviate suffering could possibly shorten life, the professionals intend only to relieve the otherwise intractable symptom. They foresee that there is a possibility (a risk) that life may be shortened. But there is no reasonable basis for suggesting that they intend that life be shortened, just as no reasonable person suggests that oncologists, surgeons, anaesthetists and others who carry out risky treatments actually intend that life should be shortened as a result of adverse outcomes of that treatment.

In end of life care the law permits both potentially life-prolonging treatments and measures to alleviate otherwise intractable symptoms where there is an associated risk of shortening life, but concern is sometimes expressed about whether sedation towards the end of life (sometimes called 'terminal sedation' or 'palliative sedation therapy', see Chapter 6) is morally justifiable.

This is because society prohibits its members from intentional killing, and acts that have a foreseeable effect of causing death may also be culpable. The prohibition applies also to health care professionals, and it may be argued that it is particularly strong in their case because vulnerable patients have been entrusted to their care. It is clear in law that professionals must never intend the death of their patients. The General Medical Council (GMC) states that, according to UK case law, 'An act where the doctor's primary intention is to bring about the patient's death would be unlawful.'[1] The Mental Capacity Act explicitly stipulates in relation to decisions about life-sustaining treatment that decision-makers must not be motivated by a desire to bring about the patient's death.[2]

The situation in end of life care is further complicated by the fact that there are times when death appears to be a benefit, either from the patient's perspective, or that of the professional, or both. However, in order to uphold the protective prohibition against killing, the professional must not intend to cause death. At the same time, patients, professionals and society wish to permit the use of medication to alleviate otherwise intractable distress at the end of life, even when this may have a foreseen effect of shortening life. They also wish to permit use of risky but potentially life-prolonging treatments where foreseen adverse events could shorten life. In order to permit this, it is sometimes proposed that the doctrine of 'double effect' be invoked.

This complex and controversial doctrine draws a distinction between intended and foreseen consequences, as is normal practice in health care where the benefits of treatment are intended, whereas the harms and risks are foreseen but not intended. The doctrine permits the intended relief of otherwise intractable suffering by means of symptom control measures in that rare situation where those symptom control measures may have a foreseen effect of shortening life. The doctrine of double effect has other conditions which must be satisfied if treatment with the foreseen bad effect of shortening life is to be considered justified, but we shall not discuss them here. The doctrine cannot be used to justify euthanasia. The doctrine is discussed in detail in the online Appendix on ethical theories.

The doctrine is formulaic and detailed, and there are some problems in the clear identification of intention and of responsibility for the effects of one's acts. We discuss some problems with its use in the online Appendix. We conclude that the use of the doctrine should not be encouraged in clinical practice, although an understanding of it is useful since it is often mentioned in health care ethics and in the media. We would argue that the doctrine is not necessary (and could be unhelpful) in the great majority of clinical decisions where the relative balance of benefit to harm and risk is sufficient to justify treatment.

By contrast, the distinction between what is intended and what is foreseen is necessary and unavoidable owing to the many possible effects of pharmacological and technical treatments, and it seems to accord with the moral intuitions of most people. Although the distinction can occasionally be difficult in end of life care, the context of care by a team of professionals should encourage discussion and reflection on intentions regarding benefits, and on the possible justification of foreseen other effects. Whereas complex philosophical arguments surround the validity of distinctions between intending and foreseeing effects of one's acts, common sense has a part to play in health care ethics and this is one example where it is very important. Ordinary reasoning and moral intuition lead to the conclusion that in end of life care the aim of alleviating suffering sometimes justifies the use of measures which entail a risk of shortening life, just as the aim of prolonging life sometimes justifies the use of treatments which entail a risk of shortening it.

3.2 **Acts and omissions**

It is sometimes suggested that one bears a greater degree of accountability or responsibility for the consequences of one's actions than one's omissions. In end of life care this becomes translated into a moral distinction between withdrawing treatment (an act) and withholding treatment (an omission).

Morality is much more complex than this. Whether a decision leads to an act or an omission is not necessarily a morally relevant factor in its justification.

We are accountable for the process of decision-making, and partially for the outcomes of our decisions, whether those outcomes are the result of an act or an omission. For instance, depending on the circumstances, it may sometimes be morally wrong to commence or continue artificial hydration and at other times wrong not to use it. Moral justification rests on whether the treatment given or not given is appropriate to bring about overall benefit and accord with the patient's wishes in the circumstances.

Although the logic of this last reasoning is clear and irrefutable, health care professionals sometimes feel that it is easier to withhold a treatment than to withdraw it once started, and this applies particularly when the treatment may sustain or prolong life. Professionals feel less causally responsible and therefore less blameworthy for something they did not do (i.e. not starting/withholding treatment) as opposed to something they did do (i.e. stopping/withdrawing treatment). This can lead to a reluctance to start treatment because of the moral difficulty of stopping it if it is ineffective, or if it becomes excessively burdensome in comparison to its benefits as the disease progresses. Professionals feel more accountable for events which follow withdrawing treatment than for events which ensue when that treatment is withheld. This is illogical, but understandable.

Nevertheless, the fact is that in all health care we are as morally and legally responsible for our omissions as we are for our actions, for treatments we withhold as for those we provide or withdraw. Many life-sustaining and life-prolonging procedures are available, just as many options for symptom control are available. We are responsible for our professional choice—that is for choosing some options and discarding others. If a moral distinction is made between withholding and withdrawing treatment, for example antibiotics or artificial hydration, and it is deemed potentially more blameworthy to withdraw treatment than to withhold it, then two adverse consequences ensue.

First, doctors become unwilling to start treatment when it is appropriate, in order to avoid stopping it when it is no longer appropriate. This can result in undertreatment of patients. Second, doctors become unwilling to stop life-prolonging treatment when it is no longer appropriate, because this constitutes a withdrawal of treatment which is seen as potentially blameworthy, particularly as withdrawal may be succeeded by death. This can result in overtreatment.

It is therefore not logical or helpful to make a moral distinction between withholding and withdrawing treatment. The GMC reminds doctors that 'Although it may be emotionally more difficult for the healthcare team, and those close to the patient, to withdraw a treatment from a patient rather than to decide not to provide a treatment in the first place, this should not be used as a reason for failing to initiate a treatment which may be of some benefit to the patient. Where it has been decided that a treatment is not in the best interests of the patient, there is no ethical or legal obligation to provide it and therefore no need to make a distinction between not starting the treatment and withdrawing it.'[3] The GMC also reminds doctors that in UK law both withholding and withdrawing treatment are regarded as an 'omission' not an 'act'.[4]

Clinicians sometimes recognise that withdrawal of a treatment is ethically appropriate but the decision still generates concerns. A case analysis of transfer of a patient with end-stage motor neurone disease to a hospice setting, with planned withdrawal of non-invasive ventilation following transfer, demonstrated the basis of such concerns.[5] Despite the ventilation the patient had worsening respiratory failure. The withdrawal of ventilation generated concerns for three reasons: (i) as a specific act, it required an unavoidably explicit decision; (ii) it was likely to be associated with a short interval from withdrawal to death so that the intention could be mistaken to be the ending of life; (iii) it was an uncommon decision in the hospice. In this particular case the patient died soon after transfer with the ventilation *in situ*, the decision having been deferred because prior to transfer it had not been discussed with the patient who retained capacity. Readers interested in the clinical issues which arise partly because of the emotive nature of these decisions might wish to read this case analysis.

Clinical situations in end of life care change, often rapidly and unpredictably. What is ethically important is that treatment options are reviewed whenever the patient's clinical circumstances change, and that the treatment given is that which most accords with the patient's best interests in the present circumstance (assuming that patients who have capacity consent to it). Although there is no ethical or legal obligation to provide a treatment which is not in the patient's best interests, it can also be argued that there is no ethical justification for commencing or continuing a treatment that is not in the patient's best interests. Current British Medical Association (BMA) guidance on withholding and withdrawing life-prolonging medical treatment notes that 'When treatment fails or ceases to provide a net benefit to the patient, the primary justification for providing it no longer exists.'[6] This statement is made in the context of explanations to patients and their relatives about why a treatment will be withheld or withdrawn.

3.3 **Killing and letting die**

All people will ultimately die. If they are to be allowed die without the application of all possible interventions that hold a prospect of prolonging life, then the law and professional ethics must allow 'letting die'. 'Letting die' is the term used to describe allowing patients to die of their illness while withholding or withdrawing some potentially life-prolonging medication or procedure. 'Letting die' has to be permitted to enable humane care and medical practice; it enables patients and professionals to decide to forego those life-prolonging treatments whose harms and risks exceed the expected benefits in that patient's case, and it enables professionals to respect patients' refusal of interventions which might prolong life.

Medical technology has made it possible to prolong life much beyond the point at which death would naturally occur. It can now be said that the timing of death due to illness is for many people influenced by the extent to which those technologies and medications are employed or are withheld or withdrawn. Many people want to die without certain interventions. Indeed, surveys documented in the *End of life care strategy* report that most people would prefer to die at home,[7] despite the lack of access to certain life-prolonging treatments, such as intravenous fluids, at home. For many other patients receiving end of life care, a point is reached where the expected benefits from further attempts to prolong life are exceeded by the side-effects and burdens of treatment, including re-admission to hospital and invasive procedures. 'Letting die' is not just permitted in end of life care—it is morally required where further attempts to prolong life are not in the patient's best interests because the associated harms and risks clearly outweigh the benefits, or where the patient is refusing them. This issue is not contentious. It is spelt out in the legally sanctioned guidance on withholding and withdrawing life-prolonging treatment produced by the GMC,[8] and in similar but more detailed guidance produced by the BMA.[9]

On the other hand, society has an interest in prohibiting intentional killing (usually called murder) in all but exceptional circumstances such as war. It can be argued that because of the extent of patient vulnerability in the professional–patient relationship, there are overwhelming reasons for maintaining society's strong prohibition of killing in this relationship. In other words, killing may be something that doctors and professional carers, even more than others, should not do.

Unfortunately, the advent of technology has made the distinction between killing and letting die blurred in some cases. For example, it is sometimes argued that the act of switching off a ventilator is killing as opposed to letting die, or that withdrawal of tube feeding in the persistent vegetative state is killing as opposed to letting die. Even in these difficult examples it can and should be argued that the cause of death is the illness, not the withdrawal of life-sustaining treatment.

However, this is not the conclusion which is always reached. For example, Mary Warnock and Elisabeth Macdonald, a philosopher and a cancer specialist respectively, have argued as follows in support of physician-assisted suicide and euthanasia. They claim that 'there is no *morally* relevant difference between killing someone and allowing him to die'.[10] In support of this claim they cite examples which, to most clinicians and informed people, are straightforward situations of 'letting die', not 'killing'. They cite the case of not attempting cardiopulmonary resuscitation (CPR) at cardiac arrest in a patient with advanced malignant disease, and the case of withholding dialysis in a patient with renal failure and very severe medical problems likely to prove fatal in the near future. They then say 'The two cases exemplify decisions involving letting patients die. Morally, however, it is highly arguable that there is little difference between allowing death to take place and actively terminating life'. By the latter they mean euthanasia, for example by administration of a lethal injection. They then claim that 'doctors could find the distinction between these cases and euthanasia, both based on suffering and value of life, more difficult to draw than first appears.'[11] We do not think the distinction is difficult to draw. Moreover, it is essential to draw it. The basis of the distinction is as follows.

Morally relevant features of letting die and euthanasia are the intention behind the decision, and the cause of death. The fact that the outcome of letting die and euthanasia is death in both cases does not establish that the two decisions are morally the same.

In the case of letting die, the intention may be to respect the patient's refusal of treatment, or to avoid imposing a treatment whose associated harms and risks exceed benefit in the clinical circumstances, or both intentions may apply. By contrast, in euthanasia the intention is to cause the patient's death—the motivation being alleviation of suffering. The important fact is that the intention in letting die is completely different from the intention in euthanasia.

In the case of letting die, the cause of death is the illness, whereas in euthanasia the cause of death is a lethal injection or whatever other method of killing the patient is employed.

So it is simply illogical to state that there is no morally relevant difference between letting die and killing (euthanasia) as there clearly are morally relevant differences—of intention and causation of death.

This is obvious in the examples given by Warnock and Macdonald. Take first the example of withholding an attempt at CPR in a patient with advanced malignant disease. There is evidence that CPR has an extremely low or nil success rate in this patient group. A 2002 review of the evidence from retrospective studies led to the conclusion that 'survival after CPR is virtually nil for a patient with metastatic disease and poor performance status.'[12] So in not attempting CPR in the situation Warnock and Macdonald describe, doctors are simply withholding a treatment which has no realistic prospect of success and which is associated with invasiveness and indignity. In so doing, doctors intend to avoid inflicting on the patient a treatment which has no prospect of benefit but which entails instead only harms. The cause of death at cardiorespiratory arrest is the underlying disease, not the withholding of a treatment which would not have averted death.

Furthermore, given that there is no benefit from attempting CPR in this situation, it is extremely difficult to justify attempting it. Guidance on decision-making regarding CPR, issued in 2007 jointly by the BMA, Resuscitation Council and Royal College of Nursing, instructs that where CPR has no realistic prospect of success, in terms of re-starting the heart and breathing for a sustained period, it should not be attempted.[13]

So in the first case cited by Warnock and Macdonald it is simply irrational to assert that withholding an attempt at CPR is morally no different from killing the patient (euthanasia), since the intention and cause of death in this case are irrefutably different from intention and cause of death in euthanasia. Furthermore, the claim that there is no morally relevant difference between two acts/decisions implies that the two acts/decisions are morally the same. But no reasonable person could claim that withholding CPR in this case is morally the same as killing the patient with a lethal injection.

Similar reasoning applies to the example of withholding renal dialysis cited by Warnock and Macdonald. Renal dialysis is a burdensome treatment, and in the case described its potential to prolong life is stated to be very limited because the patient is expected to die 'in the near future' of very severe medical conditions. So the intention of withholding dialysis in this case would be to avoid imposing a burdensome treatment with very limited prospects of prolonging life. The cause of death would be renal failure or the very severe medical problems. This contrasts with euthanasia, where the intention is to cause the patient's death and the intervention (lethal injection or similar) is the cause of the patient's death.

Even eminent physicians occasionally make the same error as Warnock and Macdonald. Sir Raymond Hoffenburg, former President of the Royal College of Physicians, stated that 'The ethics of withdrawing artificial nutrition and hydration from a dying patient knowing that this will lead to death is not clearly distinct from a more deliberate positive act to end life, since in both cases the intention is the same.'[14] But the intention is *not* the same: artificial nutrition and hydration are often justifiably withdrawn from patients dying from irreversibly terminal illnesses because they can no longer provide benefit and instead are merely burdensome or even harmful. The intention is to withdraw treatment which is no longer in the patient's best interests because its harms and risks exceed any foreseeable benefit. Strangely, Sir Raymond did acknowledge that there is a legal distinction between the two decisions, which is based on clinical agreement that the artificial hydration and nutrition is no longer of any benefit, so withdrawal is legally justified. Furthermore, the cause of death is the illness of 'the dying patient' not the withdrawal of artificial hydration and nutrition.

If Warnock and Macdonald's argument were to be accepted (which in professional ethics and law it is not) then a very unfortunate conclusion would follow. For if withholding a treatment with any potential to prolong life were considered morally the same as killing, then all health care professionals who withhold such treatment (either because the patient refuses it or because of an adverse balance of benefit to harm and risk) would be acting in a way which is morally the same as killing their patients. This is a horrific conclusion. It is a conclusion which is not reached because it is contrary to both common sense and logic to assert that a health care professional who withholds or withdraws a potentially life-prolonging treatment from a patient (because the patient is refusing it or because the harms and risks outweigh the benefits) is causally and morally responsible for the patient's death. The health care professional neither causes nor intends to cause the patient's death because the cause of death is the illness. Instead, there is a professional, societal and legal consensus against Warnock and Macdonald's argument. In Section 9.1 we discuss claims of 'no morally relevant difference' or 'moral equivalence' used in arguments to support physician-assisted suicide and euthanasia. We have dealt with the issue here as it is essential that clinicians understand the morally relevant differences between letting die and killing which form the basis for consensus in both ethics and law.

Returning to the day-to-day practice of end of life care, the reality is that:

1) in some cases the distinction between killing and letting die is difficult to draw, but

2) society needs to maintain its prohibition against killing in order to protect its members, while

3) letting die has to be permitted, for example when the harms and risks of life-prolonging or life-sustaining treatment outweigh its benefits.

In order to achieve 2 and 3, the vast majority of societies prohibit euthanasia (a lethal intervention where the intention is to cause death), and permit letting die where the harms and risks of treatment outweigh its benefits or where the patient with capacity refuses treatment.

It is important to note that the distinction between killing and letting die cannot be simplified into a distinction between an act and an omission, and, even if it could be, we have established that such a distinction alone would not provide the moral justification of a decision. There are some situations in which withholding or withdrawing a life-prolonging treatment cannot be justified, even in end of life care. This is reflected in law; failing to act where one has a clear legal duty to act is culpable in law. From the moral perspective, professionals would be blameworthy if they failed to provide a potentially life-prolonging treatment where the benefits clearly outweighed the harms and risks and the patient consented to it (in the case of a patient with capacity) or where it was in the best interests of a patient who lacked capacity.

3.4 **Conclusions**

1) A decision in end of life care may result in an act or an omission; either may be blameworthy or praiseworthy. We are morally accountable for the outcomes of our omissions to the same extent that we are morally accountable for the outcomes of our acts. There is no moral difference between withholding and withdrawing treatment.

2) Letting die is permitted in certain circumstances whereas killing is prohibited. The doctrine of double effect, which relies on the moral distinction between intended and foreseen events, allows the use of measures to relieve suffering or prolong life even if those measures carry a risk of shortening life. The doctrine is not essential for moral justification of symptom relief at the end of life.

References

1. General Medical Council (2002). *Withholding and withdrawing life-prolonging treatments.* GMC, London, p. 43.
2. Department for Constitutional Affairs (2007). Mental Capacity Act 2005 Code of Practice. The Stationery Office, Norwich, p. 79.
3. GMC, op. cit. (ref. 1), para. 19.
4. GMC, op. cit. (ref. 1), p. 43.
5. Gannon C (2005). A request for hospice admission from hospital to withdraw ventilation. *J Med Ethics* **31**:383–4.
6. British Medical Association (2007). *Withholding and withdrawing life-prolonging medical treatment*, 3rd edn. Blackwell, Oxford, p. 32.
7. Department of Health (2008). *End of life care strategy.* DoH, London, p. 27
8. GMC, op. cit. (ref. 1), para. 9–11.
9. BMA, op. cit. (ref. 6), p. 3.

10. Warnock M, Macdonald E (2008). *Easeful death*. Oxford University Press, Oxford, p. 92.

11. Warnock, Macdonald, op. cit. (ref. 10), p. 95.

12. Kite S, Wilkinson S (2002). Beyond futility: to what extent is the concept of futility useful in clinical decision-making about CPR? *Lancet Oncology* 3:638–42.

13. British Medical Association, Resuscitation Council (UK), Royal College of Nursing (2007). *Decisions relating to cardiopulmonary resuscitation*. BMA, London.

14. Hoffenburg R (2006). Advance healthcare directives. *Clin Med* 6:231–3.

4

Choice and best interests: life-prolonging treatments

Three aims are central to all health care: the prolongation of life, the alleviation of suffering due to disease, and the maintenance or restoration of function. Traditionally, the 'best interests' of patients, or at least those which can be furthered by health care, have been interpreted in terms of these three aims. In this chapter we shall discuss the first aim and in the next chapter we shall be concerned with the alleviation of suffering by symptom control and to a lesser extent with the maintenance of function.

It might be objected that there is little realistic prospect of prolonging life significantly when it is appreciated that the patient is approaching the 'end of life'. But that period is of variable length, depending on the underlying illnesses from which the patient is suffering and on the emergence of symptoms and signs which indicate a poor prognosis (see Section 4.2). The *End of life care strategy* notes the following regarding trajectories of decline at the end of life:

> Some people with long term conditions remain in reasonably good health until shortly before their death, with a steep decline in the last few weeks or months of life. Others will experience a more gradual decline, interspersed with episodes of acute ill health, from which they may, or may not, recover. A third group are very frail for months or years before death, with a steady progressive decline.[1]

Writers of this strategy and other authors have reasonably concluded that there is no simple way to define the start of end of life care, and noted that the illness trajectory cannot be predicted reliably from the diagnosis.[2] For many people suffering from a chronic illness a point is reached when it is clear that they will die from their illness but it may be difficult if not impossible to estimate prognosis accurately.[3] The period designated as 'end of life care' is not well defined and perhaps not well understood,[4] but may extend from a few weeks to perhaps a couple of years, and during that time there will be a realistic possibility of significant prolongation of life by various treatments.

The issue at stake in end of life care is whether or not it is in the interests of an individual patient to continue to offer and provide treatments with limited potential to prolong life, but with inevitable associated harms (side-effects), burdens and risks. In end of life care it is easy to assume that the alleviation of symptoms should take precedence over the prolongation of life. But such an assumption is not valid, since prolongation of life, even for a short period, would be regarded by many patients and doctors as highly desirable. In end of life care, the professional responsibility is to act in the best interests of the patient when selecting treatment options which may prolong life with net benefit. The patient chooses between the options offered, but does not have unlimited 'consumer choice' because the professional has the obligation to avoid provision of treatments where harm and risk exceed benefit, and resource restrictions may also apply.[5] The appropriate offer and provision of treatment aimed at prolonging life raises complex ethical and practical issues in end of life care.

In Section 4.1 we shall deal with some preliminary issues and in the remainder of the chapter we shall consider the ethical issues as they arise at each stage of decision-making, as those stages were described in Chapter 2. We shall discuss the last stage, that of making the final decision, under two headings, first for patients with capacity and second for those without capacity for the decision in question.

In writing this chapter we are mindful of the fact that these decisions are highly emotive for patients, their relatives, and also often for health care staff, and consequently the manner in which professionals communicate with patients is extremely important.[6] Our discussion will be presented as rationally as possible and therefore risks appearing to lack compassion or to be emotionally detached. But it is precisely because this issue is so emotive that a calm and scrupulous analysis of the ethically important factors is essential in order to promote the best possible practice in decision-making. We hope that a clear appreciation of the underlying ethical principles will help to give professionals confidence in following the proper process in a sensitive and compassionate way in the emotional climate of end of life care.

4.1 Preliminary issues of ethical importance

We shall mention four preliminary issues which are relevant to decisions on life-prolonging treatments. First, it is essential that professionals understand the distinction between killing and letting die, and the lack of a moral distinction between decisions to withhold and those to withdraw such treatment, which we discuss in Chapter 3. We shall not repeat the arguments here.

Second, since in health care it is usually in the patient's best interests to attempt to prolong life, professionals sometimes wrongly assume that there is no need to justify the interventions employed in such an attempt. But there is a need to justify all health care interventions. That justification is a reasonable expectation of net benefit (i.e. an overall balance of benefit over harm and risk) from the treatment. The British Medical Association (BMA) reminds doctors of this essential principle in its guidance on withholding and withdrawing life-prolonging treatment which states that 'When treatment fails or ceases to provide a net benefit to the patient, the primary justification for continuing to provide it no longer exists'.[7] It instructs that where the treatment will not provide net benefit then 'the treatment should, ethically and legally, be withheld or withdrawn'.[8]

In other words, the onus is on the professional to justify the intervention, even if it is aimed primarily at prolonging life. The General Medical Council (GMC) spells out the grounds for this justification in a vital paragraph at the beginning of its guidance on making decisions about life-prolonging treatment:

> Doctors have an ethical obligation to show respect for human life; protect the health of their patients; and to make their patients' best interests their first concern. This means offering those treatments where the possible benefits outweigh any burdens or risks associated with the treatment, and avoiding those treatments where there is no net benefit to the patient.[9]

Thus there is an obligation not to offer or provide interventions where it is anticipated that there would be net harm and risk rather than benefit, even though the intervention might be aimed at prolonging life.

Third, there are problems of allocation of responsibility when there is an assumption that decisions about life-prolonging treatment should be made by a 'team'. This assumption is frequent in end of life care where staff from different professional groups and different specialties must work together to meet patients' needs, and most problems occur in decisions pertaining to life-prolonging treatment. For example, in the area of cancer treatment, decision-making by a multidisciplinary team (MDT) was apparently mandated by cancer standards in 2001 which stipulated that an objective of the MDT was 'to ensure that designated specialists work together effectively in teams such that decisions regarding all aspects of diagnosis, treatment and care of individual patients . . . are multidisciplinary decisions.'[10] Such statements are clearly problematic, given that the law and professional guidance indicate that an individual professional, working face-to-face with the individual patient, actually takes responsibility for health care decisions.

In its guidance on life-prolonging treatment decisions, the GMC makes it clear that whereas consensus within the team should be sought, responsibility does not actually lie with the team, and that the opinions of different team members will carry more or less weight in discussion.[11] It helpfully explains 'You should try to reach a consensus about treatment. In doing so, you should be careful to explain the participants' roles in reaching a decision and where ultimate responsibility for the decision rests. You should give careful consideration to how much weight it would be reasonable to attach to each person's views.' There is evidence that UK doctors are highly likely to consult professional colleagues about end of life decisions,[12] but significant problems of allocation of responsibility have been identified.[13] Given that virtually all responsibility for a treatment decision will devolve to one doctor (ethically and legally), the stress placed on trying to achieve consensus is puzzling—perhaps it is grounded in a belief that a consensus decision is more likely to be the best, or that consensus is in itself a benefit by promoting harmony and thus effective joint working.

The King's Fund, having consulted on this issue, found that 'Most doctors agreed that an increasingly multidisciplinary health system needed a more sophisticated and commonly understood definition of individual professional responsibilities within multidisciplinary teams.' They concluded that action was needed to 'develop a clearer statement of the role of the doctor working in an increasingly multidisciplinary clinical environment.'[14]

We discuss ethical problems of cancer multidisciplinary teams in Section 4.3.

Fourth, resources are a factor which must be considered. As technology advances, more treatments with the potential to prolong life for a limited period are emerging. But many of these treatments are very expensive, for example new palliative oncology treatments in metastatic malignancy and some interventional cardiology procedures for patients with heart failure. Cost-effectiveness is always relevant, and the less likely a drug is to achieve its aim (effect), the less cost-effective it will be overall, so drugs that benefit only a minority of recipients will be less cost-effective even if the drug itself is not very expensive. Moreover, if these treatments prolong life but do not significantly decrease morbidity and do not maintain independence, the actual costs of providing physical care during the life prolonged will be considerable. Thus in the developed world, end of life care is becoming increasingly expensive because of the costs of non-curative treatment which may extend life for longer periods.

An example helps to illustrate the moral problem. In a clinical review on the treatment of malignant melanoma it was noted that dacarbazine is the 'standard of care' as systemic treatment for metastatic melanoma. Since this condition is associated with a median survival of only six to nine months, this treatment is being given as part of end of life care. But despite being 'standard care', dacarbazine yields a response rate of only 5–15%. Furthermore, the 'response' is a delay in disease progression by 'a few months at best' and the authors admitted that 'There is no randomized evidence for an improvement in overall survival.' Thus there is no high quality evidence that life is prolonged at all, and 85–95% of patients will get no benefit and instead will endure only harms and risks. Despite these very disappointing outcomes the authors describe the effectiveness of such treatment as 'modest'.[15] We will note here that the harm done to the large majority of patients who receive no benefit but instead endure side-effects is also morally important, and there is now some recognition of this in oncology,[16] although it may not be taken into account adequately in assessment of cost-effectiveness.

There is an understandable tendency to give a very high priority to treatments that will prolong life in the context of end of life care. It might be argued that more money should be spent on trying to gain a bit more life when time is known to be limited, as many patients feel strongly that they have been 'robbed' of life if treatment is withheld for financial reasons.

It was on the basis of this argument that the National Institute for Health and Clinical Excellence (NICE), the National Health Service (NHS) rationing body, decided in 2009 that their appraisal committees should give more weight to the life-prolonging benefits of drugs for people near the end of their lives, than to that same benefit for patients not near the end of their lives.[17] The chief executive of NICE is reported as explaining that its appraisal committees may now accept 'higher incremental cost-effectiveness ratios for life-extending treatments at the end of life.'[18] The practical result is that drugs which would normally be rejected because of poor cost-effectiveness (i.e. a cost of more than £30,000 per quality-adjusted life year (QALY) gained) are likely be made available for use in patients near death, whereas treatments of similar cost-effectiveness will be denied to those not near death. Apparently patients felt the threshold for cost-effectiveness should be raised to £70,000 per QALY.[19] It is difficult to imagine how this could be funded through the NHS, given that it has been shown that the threshold of £30,000 is above what the NHS could now fund.[20,21]

The grounds cited for the change in NICE policy are that time at the end of life is more highly valued. But there is clearly an ethical problem in departing from the previous assumption by NICE that a QALY (gained by treatment) is valued the same no matter who benefits, and instead declaring that it is more highly valued in patients near the end of life. Economists from The King's Fund, which is an independent body, noted this problem.[22]

It is very questionable whether giving this priority to potentially life-prolonging treatment is justified, even in the context of end of life care. For in end of life care symptom control and adequate physical assistance and support should arguably be at least as high a priority, and perhaps a higher priority, than treatment which may extend life for a very limited period, if at all. If we assume that there must be some sort of nominal limit to overall expenditure on end of life care, very high expenditure on attempts to prolong life will result in reduced resources for symptom control and good quality nursing care. NICE has acknowledged this problem of opportunity costs,[23] and has declared that it will monitor whether the anticipated survival gains are realized when these very expensive drugs are used in NHS routine practice.[24]

It may be argued that a potential solution to the moral and financial problems of funding very expensive potentially life-prolonging treatments is to permit patients to pay for them themselves, so 'topping up' the funding available from a taxation- or insurance-funded health service. Within the UK, following consultation and debate,[25,26] it was decided in 2008 that patients should be able to receive standard NHS care and then pay 'top up' costs to fund expensive non-curative oncology treatments which the NHS will not fund because their cost-effectiveness falls below the NICE threshold.[27] Clearly, all patients have to be informed that these very expensive treatments exist, even though they may have to fund them personally.[28] It is predictable that patients who cannot fund such expensive treatments personally will be distressed and may regard themselves as 'unjustly deprived' of extra life which wealthier patients can gain. Allowing such 'top ups' to other health care funded by a state or insurance system remains morally problematic.

Since resource allocation systems vary so much from country to country we have concluded that it is not helpful to have a lengthy discussion about resource allocation. We hope instead to point out the following: first, that the costs of end of life care must include the costs of treatments which are not curative and which have only a limited potential to extend life; second, that there is a moral responsibility to distribute publicly funded benefits of end of life care justly, and that the issue of cost-effectiveness is a legitimate and necessary ethical consideration; third, that some method of rationing/resource allocation is essential to minimize injustice in the distribution of benefits funded by state or insurance systems. Those charged with the distressing and difficult task of rationing/resource allocation should be open about their decision-making processes, and every member of society will need to understand that other members do not have a limitless duty to fund life-prolonging treatment, especially in the context of end of life care where the potential to extend life is very limited. Where life-prolonging treatment is funded by the state via taxation, or by independent insurance companies, the choices available to individual patients will inevitably and rightly be limited by the necessary rationing process—neither governments nor other members of society are to blame for this reality. Where life-prolonging treatment in end of life care is publicly funded, 'consumer choice' as described in Chapter 1 is not an option from a moral or practical point of view.

4.2 **Understanding the clinical problem**

It is obviously important at the outset to know as much as possible about the prognosis of the illness. But prognosis cannot be estimated accurately. Evidence from studies with patients with cancer has shown that doctors are generally poor at predicting prognosis and tend towards over-optimism.[29] Estimates of time the patient will survive (with advanced cancer) have accuracy of only 25%, whereas predictions of the percentage chance of surviving to a certain time have 50–75% accuracy.[30] Reviewers of prognostic tools for estimating survival time in palliative care concluded that further validation of existing tools is needed in different patient populations.[31,32] It is a matter of ethical importance that professionals are mindful of this uncertainty when taking this factor into account in decisions.

An alternative approach is to focus not only on estimating the length of time which the patient might live but also on trying to predict increasing need for support as the patient's condition deteriorates. This was recommended in the UK when in 2008 'Prognostic Indicator Guidance' was issued at national level.[33] It gives clinical prognostic indicators in an attempt to estimate when patients are in the last year of life, and the indicators also serve to alert clinicians to actual or impending need for more input from health care services. The guidance does state that the clinical indicators are only indicators and must be interpreted with clinical judgement for each individual patient.

Whereas knowing about the illness and treatment possibilities is part of the science of understanding the clinical problem, the art is gaining an understanding of the particular patient's perception of the illness including prognosis, of the patient's attitude to further treatment measures including attempts to prolong life, and of other goals and priorities. This information is relevant when selecting treatment options. It is also helpful to identify early on the patient's preferences regarding disclosure of prognostic information, since there is great variation between patients in this regard.[34] We shall return to this latter ethically complex issue in Section 4.4.i.

4.3 **Selecting treatment options that offer a prospect of net benefit**

The first important issue is the location of responsibility for deciding which treatments will be offered. Our previous discussion on decision-making and

MDTs is relevant here. It emerges from professional guidance that either a consultant or a GP, depending on who will be administering the treatment, will bear responsibility for the decision, as we indicated in the previous discussion about teams. In relation to life-prolonging treatments the GMC advises that as the consultant or GP responsible for the decision:

> You must identify appropriate treatment options based on up to date clinical evidence about efficacy, side effects and other risks, referring to any relevant clinical guidelines on the treatment and management of the patient's condition, or of patients with similar underlying risk factors. You must reach a considered judgement on the likely clinical and personal benefits, burdens and risks, for the particular patient, of each of the treatment (or non-treatment) options identified.[35]

This guidance is clear and also emphasizes the need to consider both what is known about the illness and treatment in general, via evidence and guidelines, and the individual factors that are of importance in the particular case, including risk factors in this case and the patient's more personal goals and priorities. It summarizes the basis for the selection of treatment options and it explicitly includes the option not to pursue further treatments aimed at prolonging life.

But where decisions about treatment for cancer patients are concerned, this solution has been rejected in the UK, as we noted in Section 4.1. Instead, every patient is discussed in an MDT meeting and following discussion a decision is supposed to be made by the MDT regarding the treatment the individual patient should receive.[36] In reality, the only decision that could be reached by the MDT is what treatment options the patient should be offered, on the basis of reasonable expectation of benefit over harm and risk. Although this practice was introduced to bring all the relevant experts together and in the hope of improving the quality of decision-making, it is undoubtedly morally problematic and, as we have noted, it is contradictory to professional guidance issued by bodies such as the GMC.

Ironically, attempts to make treatment decisions in the MDT setting can adversely affect patient care because the team setting can effectively remove explicit individual professional responsibility for the patient's welfare and follow-up. This adverse consequence was pointed out in a 'Personal View' paper in which the author concluded that 'Clearer ownership of patients should minimize oversights generated by ever expanding teams and should improve continuity of care. An explicit responsibility for ongoing and thorough assessment should prevent everyone retreating behind specialist remits.'[37] The morally important point here is that explicit allocation of responsibility to professionals as individuals acts in practice as a safeguard for patients, since it is at least clear who is responsible for their care. Attempts at 'team decision-making' can inadvertently remove that safeguard.

Having discussed the issue of responsibility in relation to treatment option selection, we shall move on to explore a different ethical issue, namely the extent to which the patient's values and priorities should sway the crucial professional judgement about which treatments hold sufficient prospect of net benefit to justify offering them to the patient. An example from the context of palliative chemotherapy for metastatic cancer illustrates the problem in the context of end of life care.

Evidence from research on the priorities of patients with metastatic cancer was helpfully collated by Dr Jane Maher (an oncologist) and Dr Daniel Munday (a consultant in palliative medicine).[38] They noted that evidence from studies from several countries over the past 20 years suggests that patients with metastatic cancer accept lower chances of benefit and higher risks of severe side-effects than would be accepted by matched healthy controls or healthcare professionals. But what is not clear is why patients accept treatment with such high risks in return for low benefit. The ethical question which results from these observations is whether professionals should be willing to offer treatments where they personally judge that harm and risk do exceed the foreseeable benefit, on the grounds that we know some patients would find still the balance acceptable.

Munday and Maher offer evidence-based explanations as to why patients might apparently wish to receive treatments with high risks and low benefits. They noted that whereas most patients say they want full information about diagnosis and prognosis, they do not always receive such information from oncologists, and so the patients may well be accepting treatment on the basis of false impressions about prognosis and the possible benefits of the chemotherapy. They cited a study of oncology consultations which showed that the information given about potential survival benefit which could be expected from treatment was mostly vague or was not given at all, even after a patient's explicit request for that information.[39] They also noted that chemotherapy may be offered to maintain hope, or because oncologists feel a need to do something active even if patients are unlikely to benefit, or because of a reluctance to confront the issues that surround dying.

What is ethically important here is that none of these explanations could serve as a justification for offering treatment options where the professional judges that the harm and risk would clearly outweigh the expected (limited) benefit. Patients are very vulnerable in the end of life situation, and some will accept any treatment offered which has any chance of prolonging life, even for a short time. In our view it is part of the professional responsibility to offer only those treatment options where there is a reasonable expectation of benefit in excess of harms and risks. In end of life care, an ethically important part of the professional role is to protect the patient from sustaining overall harm as a result of the pursuit of attempts to prolong life, where that life is inevitably coming to an end.

Evidence has been published which demonstrates that some treatments have been provided when expert independent assessors subsequently judged that they were clinically inappropriate, for example tube feeding in advanced dementia,[40] and percutaneous endoscopic gastrostomy (PEG) and other endoscopic procedures in seriously ill patients.[41] Such publications may help to reduce such clinically inappropriate treatments, and may increase awareness of the correct decision-making process. Similarly, new guidance on attempting cardiopulmonary resuscitation (CPR) instructs professionals not to offer this procedure to patients for whom it has no realistic prospect of success.[42] We discuss decisions relating to CPR in 7.11.

Careful reading of current consensus guidance on life-prolonging treatment reveals that the selection of treatments to be offered is the responsibility of the professional. The patient's own views about the weight or priority to give to any benefits, burdens or risks come into play only when choosing between the options offered.[43] Once again, choice is available in the ordinary sense, but not in the sense of 'consumer choice' which we described in Chapter 1.

Having said this, we must note that the professional will have learned something of the patient's priorities at the stage of 'understanding the clinical problem' described above. Professionals will rightly take these into account when selecting treatment options, whereas the actual decision about what should be offered remains a matter of professional judgement and responsibility.

4.4 Making the final decision with patients who have capacity

As we explained in Section 2.3, it is absolutely essential, if there is any doubt about the patient's capacity for the specific decision, that capacity is assessed and a judgement made on whether or not the patient has capacity for that decision. Information relevant and necessary for a decision regarding life-prolonging treatment is often complex, so in order to have capacity for the decision a patient must be able to understand, retain and weigh up this significant amount of necessary information. In this section we shall discuss decision-making for patients who have capacity—readers may wish to refer back to Section 2.4 regarding the decision-making process for these patients.

4.4.i Disclosure of information

Ideally, the professional who will take responsibility for providing the treatment should be the person who presents the patient with the treatment options and who explains the potential benefits, harms and risks of each option. But this is not always what happens in practice. The situation often arises where an initial discussion takes place between a senior doctor and the patient but the patient actually consents to or (rarely) refuses the intervention in a subsequent discussion with a specialist nurse or junior doctor. From an ethical perspective it is essential that the patient is given consistent and adequate information, and that whoever finally seeks the patient's consent has the necessary knowledge base to provide this and to answer any questions.

In the context of offers of potentially life-prolonging treatment in end of life care, the issue of how much information to disclose frequently gives rise to ethical problems and sometimes to disagreement between professionals. We discuss the general issue of giving information in Section 2.4.i and conclude that there is an ethical (and a legal) obligation to disclose serious adverse outcomes, and to disclose a significant possibility that harm could exceed benefit or that the treatment may not achieve its desired aim.

In Section 2.4.i we noted that consensus professional guidance on consent stipulates that patients must be given the information that they 'want or need'. So the obligation to give information which patients 'need' persists even when they are reluctant to receive it. It is important to bear this in mind in relation to offers of potentially life-prolonging treatment in end of life care, because the benefits of such treatment are often very limited and the harms and risks significant. Informing patients about any additional benefits in terms of symptom relief is not usually ethically problematic, and we discuss those problems which do arise in Chapter 5.

Information about the potential survival benefit resulting from the treatment is clearly crucial to a patient's decision regarding whether or not to accept further treatment. But this information is logically linked to information about the prognosis without treatment, because what the patient needs to know is what *difference* the treatment offered might make. Information about survival benefit logically entails information about prognosis of the illness without the treatment; it is reasonable to argue that patients 'need' information about the prognosis of the illness in order to put into context the amount of extra life which might be gained by the treatment. But this crucial link, between knowledge of the prognosis and knowledge of the potential extension to that prognosis by the treatment, creates difficult ethical problems and not surprisingly some controversy.

The most significant ethical problem relates to the question of whether realistic information about prognosis should be provided only if the patient actually wants it, or whether it ought to be provided even to those who do not want it, on the grounds that they 'need' it to make a decision based on a realistic understanding of survival benefit. It is important to note that in this discussion we are focusing on the ethical requirement to give information to enable patients to make an adequately informed decision about treatment—we are not discussing the separate issue of how much information patients should be given about prognosis *per se.*

Evidence from research with patients who have advanced cancer indicates that patients 'want' different amounts of information about prognosis. A recent review of patients' preferences for prognostic information is helpful in informing us of the range of 'wants'.[44] (What it cannot, of course, tell us is what information those patients 'need' and so ought to be given, independent of whether or not they 'want' it.) The review showed that all patients wanted honesty, and the vast majority wanted some broad indication of their prognosis, but that preferences for quantitative information were more varied. Realistic awareness of prognosis yielded some benefits including enhanced control and end-of-life planning, whereas lack of awareness was associated with significant negative consequences, leading to the conclusion that realistic awareness of prognosis is, in general, a desirable objective for this patient group. Alongside a desire for honesty and realism, a universal desire for hope to be maintained was found. Not surprisingly, for some patients maintaining hope for their goal was irreconcilable with receiving detailed or unequivocal information about prognosis. The authors of the review did acknowledge that it is arguably necessary to give realistic information about prognosis for the purposes of decision-making, and they commented that consideration needs to be given as to how that information is imparted. The authors concluded that 'Professionals have a responsibility to provide information to patients, but also to respect the need to maintain some ambiguity about the future, if that is a patient's wish. Therefore, prognostic discussions necessitate careful, individualized assessment . . . .' Their review found that many patients do not achieve a realistic understanding of their prognosis and that they are prone to overoptimism.

The findings of the above study support attempts to bring patients to a realistic understanding of their prognosis (even aside from decision-making), as it indicates that patients benefit from being given realistic information sensitively, particularly when combined with explanation and negotiation of information needs. By contrast, harms have been identified as a consequence of lack of realistic understanding of prognosis.

Generic professional guidance does not go into detail on this particular issue. But, as we have noted, the guidance on consent does stipulate that patients 'must' be given information that they 'want' or 'need' about the potential benefits, risks and burdens, and the likelihood of success, for each treatment option offered.[45] We would argue that in end of life care, where the benefits in terms of extension of life are limited and the likelihood of achieving that benefit is often low (or very low), and where the harms, burdens and risks are significant, patients do in fact 'need' to be given realistic information about prognosis and the likelihood and magnitude of any prolongation of life via treatment.

More harm may be done by withholding information about prognosis and survival benefit than by disclosing it. Lack of realistic awareness of prognosis has been associated with negative consequences in itself. Furthermore, lack of a realistic understanding of how little some treatments can achieve may lead patients to make choices that do not truly reflect their own values and priorities; patients may then accept a burdensome treatment with very limited prospect of benefit which they would have rejected had they been better informed. These points were made in a well-referenced paper in the *European Journal of Cancer*.[46] The issue of patients (or their families) raising substantial sums of money to pay for drugs not available through the NHS is also relevant, since they (as paying 'consumers') ought to be given accurate and adequate information about what they are buying. It is also possible that patients might reject a treatment because of excessive pessimism, which they would have accepted if they had understood its benefits more fully.

Where patients show reluctance to accept information about the likelihood and magnitude of prolongation of life at the initial discussion the decision should be delayed, if possible, to allow further discussion to occur together with an explanation as to why the patient should consider the information. Studies have demonstrated the importance for patients of individualized assessment of patient's preferences for information and pacing of that information,[47,48] but these factors must be weighed against the potential disadvantages to patients of delaying decisions in order to give information in a paced manner, which usually means in successive consultations.

There is evidence that patients are not being given realistic information about the potential benefits of palliative chemotherapy (see ref. 32 cited in Section 2.4.i). In addition, a qualitative observational study of information given to patients by oncologists about palliative chemotherapy showed that in most consultations discussion about the potential survival benefit was vague or non-existent.[49] These findings are of moral concern. Similar research for other terminal illnesses might well prove equally valuable in assessing current practice and then working to improve disclosure. But it may be that, despite all the professional guidance on giving patients information which is necessary for an adequately informed decision, there is still an institutional reluctance in the health service to be honest about how little some treatments can achieve in the context of end of life care.

One explanation for inadequate disclosure is lack of time;[50] with continuing financial constraints on staff time, combined with more complex treatment decisions and emphasis on patients being seen on time in clinics, this situation is likely to worsen. Other authors have observed that as patients become more ill their preferences for information diverged from those of their families—the patients wanted less prognostic detail but families wanted more and often talked to professionals on their own,[51] a situation often encountered in clinical practice. Even if patients consent to disclosure to relatives, thus resolving the issue of potential breach of confidentiality, the problem of not disclosing to patients the information they need for decision-making remains. There are probably multiple reasons for inadequate disclosure of prognostic information and the survival benefits of treatment, including a desire not to distress patients with bad news and to try to maintain hope. But these reasons are explanations, and in our view they cannot serve as justifications for withholding this crucial information in end of life care. On the other hand, a trend towards patients being seen as consumers who have 'the right to knowledge about their treatment' may increase disclosure,[52] especially if patients are paying for treatment as a 'top up' to publicly funded health care.

Aside from information about survival benefit, it is also important to judge whether a patient ought to be given information about how a life-prolonging treatment may alter the course of the illness and the mode of death, in order that the patient can make those choices which are possible in relation to the course of the illness. Clinical examples help to illustrate the nature of this professional judgement.

Patients with motor neurone disease have a very variable course to their illness and functional loss varies in nature and in the order in which it occurs. Patients often face choices about whether or not to commence hydration/feeding via a gastrostomy tube, and non-invasive ventilation. Discussions about tube feeding and hydration should include information about the likely development and prognosis of the illness; patients need to know that whereas this treatment may alleviate symptoms it will sadly not improve function, it will not prevent pneumonia or respiratory failure which so often cause death in this illness and, if there is already significant respiratory failure, it may not greatly prolong life. Discussions about non-invasive ventilation should include explanations about its limitations, both practically and in terms of prolonging life. This is a very distressing disease, but patients can have some control over the course of the disease and some choice about how (and possibly when) they die only if they are informed about how potentially life-prolonging treatments might affect the course of the illness.

Other clinical examples can be drawn from malignant disease, where prevention of death from one cause (such as hypercalcaemia or renal failure) may lead to development of more unpleasant symptoms prior to inevitable death from another related cause. Patients with end-stage renal disease plus other terminal illness face decisions about whether or not to commence (or continue) dialysis as a life-prolonging measure.

In other words, in end of life care patients often have choices about ways of dying, and not only about how far to try to prolong life. They require information to make those choices.

It is not possible to guess which treatment options would most accord with the patient's values and priorities in these situations. If information about the ways in which the treatments may affect the course of the illness (or their harms and risks) is withheld, patients cannot possibly make that choice which is most consistent with their own values and goals. But the information about how modes of dying may be affected by treatment is complex and unpleasant, and it may also be more than some patients can face, especially if already frail and exhausted. It is a matter of professional judgement how much to divulge, and (to an extent) how much is necessary for valid consent. If disclosure has to be limited, then the patient may be asked more general questions about values and priorities so as to narrow the range of treatment options to those which are most appropriate for that individual. The patient can then be given sufficient information to consent to or refuse the treatment(s) offered.

It is obviously of the utmost ethical importance that difficult decisions such as these are led by professionals with the appropriate knowledge, sensitivity, and time available to allow adequate discussion, to provide support in decision-making and to minimize distress.

4.4.ii Patients requesting clinically inappropriate treatment

Very occasionally patients request clinically inappropriate treatment despite an explanation that it will not provide overall benefit. Sometimes the reason for the request is an understandable (but false) conviction that a particular treatment must have a good prospect of prolonging life.

As we note in Section 2.4.ii, where the clinicians are clear that what the patient is requesting is very unlikely to provide net benefit, it is ethically justifiable and appropriate for them to decline to provide the treatment. Some patients then suggest that they are willing to take the risks of serious adverse outcomes including death for a very small chance of prolonging life, and they may suggest that they will bear responsibility for an adverse outcome. They require a sensitive explanation that, in terms of ethics and law, health professionals are responsible for what they do, and that responsibility cannot be transferred to the patient. In this sense, the patient is not a 'consumer' exercising 'consumer choice'.

In their guidance on withholding and withdrawing life-prolonging treatment, the BMA advises that whereas it is not acceptable to continue to provide indefinitely treatment that is not clinically indicated and which seriously disadvantages other patients who have a better chance of survival, there may be arguments for complying with such requests for a limited period.[53] However, the opportunity cost to other patients must be a highly relevant factor in such a decision.

Occasionally in end of life care patients request that a procedure which entails life-threatening risks be carried out, but at the same time they state that if such a life-threatening event occurs it should not be treated, so that they may die. One example is the small risk of cardiorespiratory arrest due to arrhythmia during interventional cardiology for severe cardiac disease, where the arrhythmia can usually be reversed by the cardiologist. A patient who is aware that life is coming to an end may request that the intervention goes ahead, but may want to make an advance refusal of reversal of such an arrhythmia, and of CPR, during the procedure. In this situation cardiologists have to decide whether or not they are prepared to proceed with the intervention, given that the patient's advance refusal of reversal of the arrhythmia and CPR would be legally binding if correctly formulated. The current consensus guidance on decisions relating to CPR explains that in this case it may be appropriate to decline to proceed with the intervention—the decision rests with the doctor.[54] This does seem the most ethically appropriate conclusion.

4.4.iii Reviewing the decision

Very frequently it is appropriate to offer a life-prolonging treatment but also to be aware that it should be discontinued if it proves ineffective, or if the patient's condition deteriorates and the harms and risks then exceed any ongoing benefit. The GMC consensus guidance stipulates that decisions about life-prolonging treatment 'must' be reviewed at appropriate intervals or in the period of palliative or terminal care, and the doctor must determine whether the goals of treatment or the care plan remain appropriate in the patient's present condition.[55] Patients may also change their minds about treatment—a review by the clinician provides a valuable opportunity for them to consider whether or not to continue with the treatment.

It is obviously important to be honest with patients about the need for review, and to explain to them that if the treatment ceases to provide overall benefit it will be withdrawn because if continued it would result in net harm.[56] Such honesty is ethically important as it helps to prevent patients feeling abandoned, or wrongly concluding that treatment is being withdrawn when it would still be of overall benefit. Review can help to reassure patients that the professional remains concerned that whatever treatment is given is that which is best for them at the time, and it may also reassure them that they can change their mind and discontinue the treatment at any time.

4.4.iv Life-prolonging treatments and advance care planning

We discuss the ethical issues of planning in advance for future loss of capacity in Chapter 7. Here it is important to note that the information that patients with capacity ought to be given to enable them to make contemporaneous decisions should also be provided if they are wishing to express or are being asked to express preferences regarding life-prolonging treatment in a future situation where they will lack capacity. This ethically important professional responsibility is easily overlooked in the current enthusiasm for advance care planning discussions, advance statements and advance decisions to refuse treatment.

4.5 Making the final decision: patients without capacity

Making decisions about life-prolonging treatment on behalf of patients who lack capacity to decide for themselves is notoriously difficult, and the patients concerned are very vulnerable. Therefore, in addition to professional guidance, laws may stipulate the decision-making process. In Section 2.5 we outline the issues that laws governing such decisions must cover, and as an example we describe the decision-making process stipulated by the Mental Capacity Act 2005 which applies in England and Wales. The decision-making process for potentially life-prolonging treatments is essentially the same as for other treatment and care decisions.

In the following discussion we do not address the issues pertaining to life-prolonging or life-sustaining treatment in patients whose condition is essentially stable and in whom a deterioration is not clearly foreseen. This would include patients who are stable but dependent on hydration and nutrition via gastrostomy (PEG) tubes, perhaps following a stroke, and patients who are in a persistent vegetative state or similar condition. Decision-making for these patients is undoubtedly very difficult, but the relevant clinical circumstances are very different from those of end of life care.

4.5.i **Special features of decision-making regarding life-prolonging treatment**

Laws governing decision-making for patients lacking capacity may make provision for patients to make advance refusals of life-prolonging treatment. If a patient has made such a refusal, and if it is valid and applicable in the circumstances and its formulation meets the requirements of the relevant law, it will generally be legally binding. In such a case the patient has made the decision to refuse the treatment, and therefore professionals will not be required to make a decision on the patient's behalf. The problems of assessing validity and applicability of advance decisions to refuse treatment, and of advance statements, are considered in detail in Chapter 7.

Some laws, for example the Mental Capacity Act, enable a patient who retains capacity to appoint someone (an attorney) to make healthcare decisions on the patient's behalf if the latter should lose capacity. The attorney will consent to or refuse treatment on behalf of the patient (according to the scope of authority the patient has given). Under the Mental Capacity Act the attorney's decision must be based on his/her judgement of the patient's best interests, but laws in other countries may stipulate that it should be a substitute judgement (see Section 2.5). Attorneys clearly bear a major responsibility when they are entrusted with decisions pertaining to life-prolonging treatment. As they are deciding in lieu of the patient they will require the same information as the patient ought to have received if the patient had capacity. They may also require, and should be offered, the same support as a patient might require in decision-making.

Since patients who lack capacity are in a position of great vulnerability, professional ethics and law may stipulate extra protection for them in relation to decisions about life-prolonging or life-sustaining treatment. The Mental Capacity Act has two protective stipulations—both are ethically necessary and important.[57]

The first is that the decision-makers 'must not be motivated by a desire to bring about the person's death for whatever reason, even if this is from a sense of compassion.'[58] Thus the decision must be based on whether the treatment is in the patient's best interests, and not on a desire that the patient should die, or on the view that death would be better for the patient (or others).

The second stipulation is that decision-makers should not make assumptions about the patient's quality of life. This implies that no attempts should be made to assess or judge the patient's quality of life. The BMA explains the moral reasons behind this; it notes that the term 'quality of life' can be problematic and ambiguous and that 'when used by others in relation to people lacking capacity . . . the term can be interpreted to imply that some people's lives are less valued.' They stress that the doctor's role is not to determine the value or worth of the patient's life, but instead is to determine whether the proposed treatment measures would gain for patients 'a way of living they would be likely to consider acceptable, despite any side-effects or disadvantages of treatment'. Although they conclude that use of the concept of quality of life is now unavoidable, they warn that assessment tools for quality of life should not be used when best interests judgements are being made.[59]

To this we would add that it is impossible for one person to know, or to assess (much less measure) the quality of another person's life. Furthermore, there is no coherent shared understanding of what factors are included in quality of life. We developed these arguments in a previous work.[60]

This stipulation puzzles those health care professionals who have become accustomed to the idea that a judgement about the patient's quality of life made by someone other than the patient is a legitimate and perhaps even essential factor in these decisions. Sometimes relatives of patients similarly consider that their judgement of the patient's quality of life should be taken into account.[61] In the UK, professional guidance and law acting together are trying to prevent professionals from using assumptions, assessments or judgements about the patient's quality of life in decisions about life-prolonging treatment, and to prevent notions of the value of the patient's life, or the value of life to the patient, being similarly used.

4.5.ii Consulting the patient

Even when they lack capacity for the decision, patients may still be able to express wishes, feelings, beliefs or values which are relevant to the decision and so must be taken into account. It is important to note interventions which the patient indicates are distressing.

Where patients do not appear to want an intervention, but lack capacity to make the decision, it must be remembered that they are not actually making a considered *refusal* of the treatment. It will sometimes be in a patient's best interests to pursue a treatment which the patient does not appear to want, such as antibiotics that have a good prospect of success when a patient has become confused as a result of an infection.

Advance statements or preferences recorded with the patient's consent must obviously be taken into account. A preference not to return to hospital is clearly important in treatment decisions. We consider the associated ethical issues in Chapters 7 and 8.

4.5.iii Consulting those close to the patient

In Section 2.5 we describe the process of consultation with the family and close friends of the patient in order to gain information about the patient's wishes, feelings, beliefs and values and the factors which the patient would consider if he/she had been able to do so. Family members will be asked what they think the patient would have wanted, as well as their views about what would be in the patient's best interests. If the patient has been in residential care, or has been reliant on professional carers at home, it is likely to be appropriate to ask their opinion on these issues as well. Such consultation raises issues of confidentiality which we discuss in Section 2.5.

Those close to the patient who are consulted do bear a significant responsibility in the decision-making process (although they will not bear responsibility for the final decision). This can be onerous for them, and it is important that they are encouraged and given support to consider the issues carefully. Some may feel enduring guilt, regardless of how conscientiously they take part in the process. It is important that they understand that they are not responsible for the final decision, since this understanding may reduce the likelihood of later feelings of guilt or family disputes and recriminations.

Patients who lack capacity and have no friends or family members whom it is appropriate to consult are in a particularly vulnerable position, and professionals charged with decision-making on their behalf may lack information about the patient's values and priorities. Laws and professional guidance may try to safeguard their interests by advising or requiring the use of independent advocates. For example, the Mental Capacity Act stipulates that if a serious medical treatment decision is at stake, such as a decision about life-prolonging treatment, an independent advocate must be appointed.[62] The advocate is effectively functioning as a substitute family member in so far as this is possible, finding out about the patient's wishes and feelings, beliefs and values, then representing these to the decision-maker to assist in making the best interests judgement. The advocate is not a decision-maker. Clearly, in emergency or urgent situations time does not permit the appointment and involvement of advocates—professionals then make treatment decisions based on patients' best interests.

4.5.iv The basis of the final decision

Laws and professional guidance are likely to stipulate that the basis of the final decision must be the patient's best interests. This is the case in the UK and via the Mental Capacity Act. Sometimes the patient's best interests may conflict with those of family members, but in the case of life-prolonging treatment it is absolutely clear from an ethical perspective that the decision must be based only on the patient's interests.

Health care professionals sometimes have concerns that family members may be influenced by their own interests when considering and reporting both what the patient might have wanted and what, in their view, is in the patient's best interests. But to an extent it just is human nature to be influenced by one's own interests, and this complication to the process is ineradicable. Professionals have no alternative but to rely on the honesty of those close to the patient; although they will report on the patient's wishes, feelings, beliefs and values, and present their view on what is in the patient's best interests, it is actually the professionals who will make the decision.

Occasionally relatives request attempts to prolong life which are obviously not in the best interests of the patient; professional guidance, supported by law in the UK, has then ruled that professionals should not comply with the request.[63]

In cases of conflict of views between the family and professionals about the patient's best interests, it can be very helpful to seek a second opinion.[64] Ideally this should be contributed by a professional who is as independent as possible from the decision-maker. If there is enduring uncertainty about the decision, or enduring conflict, the relevant law covering decisions for patients who lack capacity may provide a special court to make the decision. Under the Mental Capacity Act this is called the Court of Protection.

4.5.v Reviewing the decision

As in the case of patients with capacity it is essential to review decisions. Those close to the patient should be informed that this will occur, and they are likely to be reassured by this process, in the same way that a patient with capacity may be.[65]

4.6 Conclusions

1. In the context of end of life care, treatment aimed at prolonging life may still be in the best interests of the patient. But the provision of such treatment must be justified by a reasonable expectation of benefit exceeding the harms, burdens and risks.

2. The professional responsibility for the decision will lie with one health care professional; that individual will take into account the views of other team members.

3. As the cost of non-curative treatments aimed at prolonging life increases, resource constraints are likely to limit the range of treatments available from publicly funded health care systems. Cost-effectiveness and fairness are legitimate and necessary considerations in the allocation of finite resources.

4. The professional role includes the selection of treatment options which it is justifiable to offer to the patient with capacity, or consider for a patient

lacking capacity; that justification rests on a reasonable prospect of net benefit in the circumstances of the individual patient.

5. Patients (or the family of the patient where the latter lacks capacity) ought to be informed about the likely prognosis with and without the treatment aimed at prolongation of life. They should also receive an explanation of how the treatment may alter the course of the illness and the mode of death, if they are willing to confront these issues.

6. Patients who lack capacity for the decision may still be able to express relevant wishes, feelings, beliefs or values. Any statement pertaining to these factors, which they made prior to loss of capacity, should be taken into account.

7. Decisions about potentially life-prolonging treatment made on behalf of patients who lack capacity must be based on the patient's best interests, and not on the interests of family members. Such decisions should not be based on judgements made by others about the patient's quality of life.

References

1. Department of Health (2008). *End of life care strategy*. DoH, London, p. 45.
2. Strandburg T (2008). Cardiovascular disease and cancer in very old age. *BMJ* 337:a2521.
3. DoH, op. cit. (ref. 1), p. 51.
4. Shipman C, Gysels M, White P, *et al.* (2008). Improving generalist end of life care: national consultation with practitioners, commissioners, academics, and service user groups. *BMJ* 337:a1720.
5. Elwyn G, Buetow S, Hibbard J, Wensing M (2007). Respecting the subjective: quality measurement from the patient's perspective. *BMJ* 335:1021–2.
6. Smyth JF (2009). Communication as important as cure. *European Journal of Cancer* 45:6–7.
7. British Medical Association (2007). *Withholding and withdrawing life-prolonging medical treatment*, 3rd edn. Blackwell, Oxford, p. 32.
8. BMA, op. cit. (ref. 7), p. 3.
9. General Medical Council (2002). *Withholding and withdrawing life-prolonging treatments*. GMC, London, para. 9.
10. Department of Health (2001). *Manual of cancer services standards*. DoH, London, p. 28.
11. GMC, op. cit. (ref. 9), para. 56.
12. Seale C (2006). Characteristics of end-of-life decisions: survey of UK medical practitioners. *Palliative Medicine* 20:653–659.
13. The King's Fund (2008). *Understanding doctors; harnessing professionalism*. The King's Fund, London, pp. 46–49.
14. The King's Fund, op. cit. (ref. 13), p. 51–52.
15. Thirlwell C, Nathan P (2008). Melanoma part 2: management. *BMJ* 337:a2488.

16. Smyth, op. cit. (ref. 6), p. 6.

17. National Institute for Health and Clinical Excellence (2008). *Social value judgements: principles for the development of NICE guidance*. NICE, London.

18. Kmietowicz Z (2009). NICE lifts cost limit on drugs to improve access to end of life treatments. *BMJ* **338**:b3.

19. White C (2008). NICE to confer on taking more account of patients' views. *BMJ* **337**:a2211.

20. Appleby J, Devlin N, Parkin D (2007). NICE's cost effectiveness threshold. *BMJ* **335**:358–9.

21. Collier J (2008). Parliamentary review asks NICE to do better still. *BMJ* **336**:56–7.

22. Appleby J, Maybin J (2008). Topping up NHS care. *BMJ* **337**:a2449.

23. O'Dowd A (2008). Watchdog set to reject four kidney cancer drugs for NHS. *BMJ* **337**:a1262.

24. Kmietowicz, op. cit. (ref. 18).

25. Gubb J, Bloor K (2008). Should patients be able to pay top-up fees to receive the treatment they want? *BMJ* **336**:1104–5.

26. Donaldson C (2008). Cancer drug top-ups: can we kill the zombie for good? *BMJ* 2008;**337**:a578.

27. Richards M (2008). *Improving access to medicines for NHS patients*. Department of Health, London.

28. GMC, op. cit. (ref. 9), para. 25.

29. Glare P, Virik K, Jones M, *et al.* (2003). A systematic review of physician's survival predictions in terminally ill cancer patients. *BMJ* **327**:195–201.

30. Glare P, Sinclair C, Downing M, Stone P, Maltoni M, Vigano A (2008). Predicting survival in patients with advanced disease. *European Journal of Cancer* **44**:1146–56.

31. Lau F, Cloutier-Fisher D, Kuziemsky C, *et al.* (2007). A systematic review of prognostic tools for estimating survival time in palliative care. *Journal of Palliative Care* **23**:93–112.

32. Glare, Sinclair, Downing, Stone, Maltoni, Vigano, op. cit. (ref. 30), 1146–56.

33. Gold Standards Framework Centre (2008). *Prognostic indicator guidance*. Available at http://www.goldstandardsframework.nhs.uk (accessed 14 January 2009).

34. Innes S, Payne S (2009). Advanced cancer patients' prognostic information preferences: a review. *Palliative Medicine* **23**:29–39.

35. GMC, op. cit. (ref. 9), para. 36–7.

36. Department of Health (2001). *Manual of cancer services standards*. Department of Health, London, pp. 22–41.

37. Gannon C (2005). Will the lead clinician please stand up? *BMJ* **330**:737.

38. Munday DF, Maher EJ (2008). Informed consent and palliative chemotherapy. *BMJ* **337**:a868.

39. Audrey S, Abel J, Blazeby JM, Falk S, Campbell R (2008). What oncologists tell patients about survival benefits of palliative chemotherapy and implications for informed consent: qualitative study. *BMJ* **337**:a752.

40. Monteleoni C, Clark E (2004). Using rapid-cycle quality improvement methodology to reduce feeding tubes in patients with advanced dementia: before and after study. *BMJ* **329**:491–4.

41. National Confidential Enquiry into Patient Outcome and Death (2004). *Scoping our practice.* Available at http://www.ncepod.org.uk

42. British Medical Association, Resuscitation Council (UK), Royal College of Nursing (2007). *Decisions relating to cardiopulmonary resuscitation.* BMA, London.

43. GMC, op. cit. (ref. 9), para. 41.

44. Innes, Payne, op. cit. (ref. 34), pp. 1–11.

45. General Medical Council (2008). *Consent: patients and doctors making decisions together.* GMC, London, para. 9 e.

46. Glare *et al.*, op. cit. (ref. 30), p. 1151.

47. Innes, Payne, op. cit. (ref. 34), p. 4.

48. Kirk P, Kirk I, Kristjanson J (2004). What do patients receiving palliative care for cancer and their families want to be told? A Canadian and Australian qualitative study. *BMJ* **328**:1343–7.

49. Audrey, Abel, Blazeby, Falk, Campbell, op. cit. (ref. 39), a752.

50. Fallowfield L (2001). Participation of patients in decisions about treatment for cancer. *BMJ* **323**:1144.

51. Kirk, Kirk, Kristjanson, op. cit. (ref. 48), p. 1346.

52. Morris M (2004). Informing cancer patients. *British Journal of Cancer Management* **1**:16–19.

53. BMA, op. cit. (ref. 7), p. 48.

54. BMA *et al.*, op. cit. (ref. 42).

55. GMC, op. cit. (ref. 9), para. 64.

56. BMA, op. cit. (ref. 7), p. 32.

57. Department for Constitutional Affairs (2007). Mental Capacity Act 2005 Code of Practice. The Stationery Office, Norwich, p. 65.

58. DCA, op. cit. (ref. 57), p. 79.

59. BMA, op. cit. (ref. 7), p. 8, 10.

60. Randall F, Downie RS (2006). *The philosophy of palliative care: critique and reconstruction.* Oxford University Press, Oxford, pp. 25–51.

61. Anonymous (2008). Life is for living. *BMJ* **337**:a2529.

62. DCA, op. cit. (ref. 57), pp. 179–81.

63. Dyer O (2005). Judges support doctors' decision to stop treating dying man. *BMJ* **331**:536.

64. GMC, op. cit. (ref. 9), para. 17.

65. BMA, op. cit. (ref. 7), pp. 40–41.

5

Choice and best interests: symptom control and the maintenance of function

Professionals further the best interests of their patients by pursuit of the three aims of health care, which we have noted as the prolongation of life, the alleviation of suffering and the restoration or maintenance of function. In this chapter we discuss the ethical issues which arise in pursuit of the aim of alleviation of suffering in end of life care; the aim of restoration or maintenance of function occasionally gives rise to similar issues.

Sometimes measures to alleviate suffering may also either prolong life, or may very occasionally entail a risk of shortening it—both these effects can give rise to ethical problems in clinical practice. The balance of benefit to harm and risk can also pose moral problems; since professionals bear responsibility for acting only in the best interests of their patients, they retain the obligation to avoid provision of treatments where harm and risk exceed benefit. This ethical obligation largely governs the selection of treatment options.

Sedation is sometimes used to alleviate suffering at the end of life and there is consensus on its use where patients are imminently dying. However, recently some controversy and confusion have developed round the ethics of sedation. The controversy has been created by some who say that since sedation may, in certain circumstances, hasten death it is therefore tantamount to causing the death of the patient and is therefore a form of euthanasia. From these false premises some writers draw the conclusion that euthanasia should be legalized, while others may conclude that the use of sedation should be minimized. We discuss these arguments in Section 9.1. The confusion has arisen over the term 'terminal sedation', which is open to a number of interpretations. These issues are of such importance and current interest that we discuss them separately in Chapter 6.

5.1 The basis of most moral problems in symptom control

Many patients suffer from severe symptoms in the last months of their lives, either due to the terminal illness itself or due to coexisting pathologies.

Most treatments for the relief of pain and other symptoms have some harmful side-effects which may in turn cause further symptoms, and they may also be associated with risks, particularly when an invasive procedure is undertaken. The judgement about whether the potential benefit of a treatment justifies the associated harms and risks is crucial in selecting treatment options for symptom control. Professionals bear responsibility for selecting the treatment options offered to patients with capacity, and considered for those lacking capacity, taking into account the patient's clinical circumstances and priorities.

Whereas the patient has choice in the ordinary sense (between the options offered), the patient does not have choice in the sense of 'consumer choice' because the professional remains accountable for what is provided and for safeguarding the patient from net harm.

In Section 2.2, we discussed the principles underlying the selection of treatment options, noting that treatments should be offered (or considered for patients lacking capacity) only if there is a realistic expectation that benefit will exceed harm and risk. But we must stress that although the underlying principles are clear, there can be no rigid rules to govern the individual clinical decision—the doctor must exercise clinical judgement in the particular clinical circumstances of the individual patient. That judgement is particularly necessary where there is uncertainty about the balance of benefit to harm and risk, or where potential benefit is great but there are also significant harms or risks.

There is consensus that alleviating suffering must be a high priority in end of life care, but ethical problems arise from the difficulties of balancing benefits against the harms and risks of treatment, including when (very rarely) there is a risk of shortening life. Occasionally the interests of relatives and other patients seem also to be relevant, giving rise to further difficult moral problems. Since some problems, and the process of decision-making, differ between patients with capacity and those lacking capacity we discuss them separately.

5.2 Moral problems of symptom control in patients with capacity

We have noted that the *balance* of the expected benefit (alleviating suffering) to the foreseen harms and risks determines which treatment options should be offered to patients; this could be summarized as a principle of 'proportionality'. This clinical value judgement, which is often complex and sometimes difficult, is an inescapable professional responsibility. Acting in patients' best interests requires that treatments which are likely to be futile or very unlikely to alleviate the symptom, or whose harms and risks greatly outweigh their benefits, are not offered. But where a symptom has proved intractable, significant harms and risks may be balanced by realistic potential for benefit, justifying the offer of the treatment. Resource constraints may also affect the range of treatments available.

The nature and amount of information which patients want to be given in the course of decision-making varies. We noted in Section 2.4.i that guidance from the UK General Medical Council (GMC) states that patients must be given the information that they 'want or need' in order to decide whether to consent to treatment.[1] It also stipulates that doctors 'must' give patients information about serious adverse outcomes and 'should' give information about frequently occurring but less serious side-effects or complications.[2] But we also noted that this guidance does not indicate criteria by which to judge what information is 'needed' for a decision, nor does it adequately explain what should be done when the patient does not want information, or when exhaustion makes considering information burdensome.

Furthermore, the GMC reminds doctors that before accepting patients' consent (and therefore proceeding with treatment) 'you must consider whether they have been given information they want or need, and how well they understand the details and implications of what is proposed.'[3] So the GMC appears to be stating that if information which patients 'need' is not given, consent is of very dubious validity and treatment should not proceed.

This is morally highly problematic in the context of symptom control in end of life care, where patients may be extremely weary and debilitated mentally and physically. Whilst they retain capacity, they may not actually want the amount of information about symptom control options which they 'should' be given, and perhaps not even the lesser amount which they 'must' be given. The more they are distressed and debilitated by severe symptoms, and thus the more they are in need of symptom relief, the less mental energy they may have to receive and deliberate on significant amounts of information. Some may also be very anxious about the future, and thus be rather fearful about information they perceive as more 'bad news'. It is not that the information would cause them 'serious harm', which the GMC would accept as a justification for not giving it. It is rather that exhausted and/or anxious patients may simply not want it.

The consequences of declaring consent invalid, because information which patients 'need' or 'must' be given has not been disclosed, appear to be very bad for patients. In the absence of valid consent, these very distressed and debilitated or anxious patients cannot be given the treatment which would diminish their suffering. From the ethical perspective, this outcome is intuitively unacceptable. Furthermore, it appears that the process of joint decision-making and consent, which has evolved to protect patients, has in this particular situation severely disadvantaged them. There are two potential solutions which can be considered.

The first would be to encourage patients to express preferences regarding how much information is given to them and to agree to withhold information which they do not want. Professionals could then ascertain the patient's wishes and feelings, beliefs and values and, taking these into account, propose a treatment which most accorded with the patient's best interests. This treatment would then be provided, assuming that the patient agreed to it. We acknowledge in Sections 2.4.i and 2.4.iii that some authors, including philosophers, have suggested that patients should be allowed to choose the extent to which they are involved in decision-making. Professionals could then be allowed discretion regarding what information was disclosed. We would support this solution, especially in the context of symptom control in end of life care, where the great majority of treatments are not excessively harmful or risky and the clinical priority is alleviation of suffering. But we are not certain how law (in the UK or elsewhere) or bodies governing professional standards would judge this solution.

The second solution is to consider carefully what would constitute a 'serious adverse outcome' for a patient in the context of end of life care, for it is only outcomes in this category which professional guidance clearly states 'must' be disclosed. Clinical examples help us to consider which serious adverse outcomes due to symptom control measures could be foreseen, and then we can judge whether there is a moral imperative to inform patients about them.

The most obvious serious adverse outcome is death. It is very difficult to imagine a clinical situation in which a symptom control measure could actually cause death, assuming proper clinical practice in terms of prescribing. Major opiate overdoses could theoretically cause death through respiratory depression, but such an event is much more likely to be due to accidental overdose, and with proper prescribing practice it would not occur. Therefore it is not a foreseen outcome, and we do not warn patients about the adverse effects of large overdoses of medications prescribed. Non-steroidal anti-inflammatory drugs (NSAIDs) can cause significant deterioration in renal function which can be hazardous for patients with pre-existing renal impairment. Therefore, if NSAIDs were being considered for a patient with significant renal impairment it does seem reasonable to assert that the patient ought to be informed of the risk of worsening renal failure, in order that the patient could decide whether, in the circumstances, the risk was worth taking for the sake of better pain relief. If the patient declined such involvement in the decision, then our first proposed solution seems the only feasible option.

One example of a symptom control measure which could hasten death is the use of sedation to relieve intractable pain and distress; if a patient is not imminently dying and requests continuous sedation so as to be rendered less aware of distress, it does seem reasonable to assert that the patient ought to be informed that such sedation could hasten death from the underlying terminal illness, or that (in extreme cases) it could cause death. This issue is discussed in Chapter 6. Another example is the use of oxygen in patients close to death with hypercapnic respiratory failure, which we discuss in Section 3.1. Such patients are likely to be already aware of the potential dangers of oxygen in their case.

Other serious adverse outcomes mentioned by the GMC,[4] and discussed in Section 2.4.i, may very occasionally occur through symptom control measures in end of life care. For example, nerve blocks could cause numbness and possibly weakness or paralysis. But it is clear that these particular adverse effects must be explained to patients as otherwise they are not in a position to decide whether to consent to the treatment or not.

The question then arises as to how much information should be disclosed about common but less serious adverse effects of symptom control measures. Clinicians making decisions with exhausted or anxious patients, who are understandably reluctant to consider much information, have to make a judgement about how much detail should be given to each patient. It is not plausible to argue that patients who do not want much information 'need' to be told about a litany of less serious adverse effects. Therefore, disclosure of these harms and risks is more a matter of professional judgement than overriding obligation.

Consideration must also be given to disclosure of potentially life-prolonging effects of interventions primarily aimed at alleviating suffering. Prolonging life is not normally considered an 'adverse effect' or 'side-effect' of treatment, so professional guidance does not cover disclosure of this effect! But, in the context of end of life care, information about such prolongation of life may be of crucial importance to patients in weighing up the effects of treatment in comparison with their own priorities. Some patients want their life prolonged but others do not—they may judge that their level of comfort or function has deteriorated to the point that they would prefer death to result from the illness earlier rather than later.

For example, the symptoms of a chest infection occurring in the very frail can be alleviated by antibiotics which may cure the infection but may well also prolong life. Patients who do not want this latter outcome may prefer to opt for other methods of symptom control such as medications to reduce secretions and alleviate dyspnoea. Patients with anaemia due to marrow failure face difficult choices in relation to continuing transfusions; transfusion may improve symptoms but for some patients it may also prolong life, and may indeed prolong it until thrombocytopenia intervenes with consequent risk of haemorrhage. Patients who have subacute intestinal obstruction with intermittent vomiting due to disseminated intra-abdominal malignancy may feel more comfortable if they receive parenteral hydration, but this measure might significantly prolong life, especially if the obstruction worsens but is not catastrophic. Such patients might not want life prolonged in the face of irreversible intestinal obstruction. If these life-prolonging effects of symptom control measures are explained to patients they can take them into account, alongside the other relevant factors in their decision.

The extent to which patients will wish to discuss these issues will vary. Discussions about possible prolongation of life will usually entail disclosure of information about prognosis, with and without the intervention under discussion, and we discuss this in Section 4.4.i. A review of evidence regarding patients' preferences for prognostic information found that:

> Although the literature indicated that most patients wanted some indication of a limited life span, some shied from the prospect of any more detailed information than that. Patients frequently identified that unwanted or uninvited information would serve to destroy hope for them, and it is therefore important that prognostic disclosure is not an active procedure undertaken by the professional, with the patient a passive recipient. It is a discussion where the function of information is negotiated and the awareness of the patient is created in the context of their own particular needs.[5]

The authors of this review concluded that 'professionals must decide how much information to give each patient and the best way of presenting it.' This is a matter of clinical judgement, and the professional responsibility for that judgement is a significant one. Professionals should consider whether a patient ought to be given an explanation of the potential life-prolonging effects of symptom control interventions, in order to help them decide whether to accept the intervention or to decline it.

5.3 Moral problems of symptom control in patients who lack capacity

In relation to ethical issues pertaining to symptom control, patients who lack capacity can be considered in two groups: those for whom death is imminent, and those who are not imminently dying but lack capacity due to problems such as diminished consciousness, confusion or mental illness.

5.3.i Moral problems when the patient is imminently dying

Patients for whom death is imminent should, whenever possible, be identified by the health care team in order to arrange for appropriate care and medications to be continuously available. Within the UK it is recommended that particular guidance, called the Liverpool Care Pathway for the Care of the Dying (LCP), is followed in order to optimize the patient's care and to promote appropriate understanding among, and support for, the patient's friends and family.[6] Physical comfort and the relief of psychological distress are the priorities of care for those who are imminently dying, and it is important not only that appropriate symptom control is given but also that ineffective and burdensome treatment is not commenced or is discontinued. These priorities are not contentious.

But it is a matter of the utmost ethical importance that the 'diagnosis of dying' is made conscientiously and that the LCP is not used inappropriately. In order to avoid such inappropriate application, criteria for use of the pathway are laid down and must be followed. They are:

All possible reversible causes for the current condition have been considered:

The multiprofessional team has agreed that the patient is dying, and two of the following may apply:–

| the patient is bedbound | . . . | semi-comatose |
| only able to take sips of fluid | . . . | no longer able to take tablets |

The pathway is designed for use only in the last few days or perhaps week of life (as the period when imminent death can be predicted varies according to the patient's clinical condition). It ought not to be used unless the multiprofessional team has made a considered clinical judgement that the patient is imminently dying.

The use of most standard interventions to alleviate symptoms in patients imminently dying is not contentious. For example, the provision of adequate analgesia, control of nausea and vomiting as far as possible, mouth care and treatment, and measures to alleviate micturition difficulties are not contentious. The benefit of controlling these symptoms at the end of life clearly outweighs the harms and risks associated with the medications when the latter are used in accordance with proper practice. The pathway includes guidance for non-specialists on proper practice in the use of medications.

As we shall mention later in the discussion on terminal sedation, the giving of medication to alleviate agitation at the end of life is also not usually contentious. The LCP guides professionals to look for signs of delirium, terminal anguish and restlessness (thrashing, plucking or twitching). If no reversible causes can be found and rectified (for example retention of urine) the pathway suggests low doses of benzodiazepines (midazolam), given initially as single injections as needed, but then by continuous subcutaneous infusion if more than three doses per day are required. Since this medication is likely to sedate the patient, the objection is occasionally raised that the sedative may decrease further the patient's ability to communicate. But the alternative of withholding sedation and leaving a dying patient in distress, for the sake of an ever-diminishing prospect of communication with others, is intuitively unacceptable. The interests of the patient are paramount in this situation; sedation which the patient needs should not be withheld or withdrawn at the request of family members who wish to try to retain communication with the patient.

By contrast, the administration of hyoscine hydrobromide to reduce respiratory secretions in unconscious patients is contentious, the reason being that such patients may not be distressed at all by the presence of secretions in the throat. If the patient is not distressed, there seems no justification for giving hyoscine, especially since it has effects which could be deleterious—it has sedative effects which may not be desired, and it causes a dry mouth and so may aggravate any oral discomfort. The primary reason for giving the hyoscine is to attempt to reduce the distress relatives may feel when hearing the 'death rattle'. This sound is caused by secretions in the throat which the patient no longer clears by coughing. So whereas the LCP recommends the use of hyoscine (or glycopyrronium, which is not sedative), it is currently not clear that this practice is ethically justifiable. UK law requires that decisions made on behalf of patients who lack capacity must be based only on the patient's best interests. If the patient is not distressed the only legal justification for the hyoscine would be evidence that the patient would have considered reducing the distress of relatives to be an important personal priority. Nevertheless, in making the best interests judgement, reducing the distress of relatives would still have to be weighed against any adverse effects of the hyoscine on the patient. An alternative, and ethically acceptable, solution would be explanation and reassurance to the family so that they did not feel distressed by the sound.

An issue which is sometimes contentious is the commencement or continuation of artificial hydration in the last few days of life. The argument used in favour of such hydration (via nasogastric or percutaneous endoscopic gastrostomy (PEG) tube, or subcutaneous or intravenous routes) is that it might alleviate thirst. The arguments against such hydration are that it may not alleviate any feelings of thirst which the patient might still perceive, that rather than 'prolonging life' it may instead 'prolong dying', that it might cause adverse effects such as increasing peripheral oedema and ascites, and that it involves treatment which is often invasive and thus possibly burdensome to the patient. It would clearly not be justifiable to insert a PEG tube or nasogastric tube in the last few days of life, but the issue of whether or not to continue hydration via tubes which are already *in situ* at the end life is inescapable.

In an attempt to establish the balance of any benefit to harm and risk in relation to artificial hydration in the context of palliative care, a Cochrane review of the literature on parenteral hydration in this context was carried out.[7] A similar review and guidance was produced by the UK Association for Palliative Medicine and was published by the National Council for Palliative Care.[8] Both groups concluded that there was little evidence overall, and that there was no conclusive evidence of benefit from artificial hydration in the last few days of life. However, there was some evidence indicating that peripheral oedema, ascites and pleural effusions were worsened by continued artificial hydration. Thus, once again, professionals must judge what is in the best interests of each individual patient, bearing in mind the patient's clinical circumstances and previous wishes, feelings, beliefs and values. The LCP appropriately prompts professionals to review interventions and to discontinue those which are inappropriate, citing intravenous fluids as an intervention requiring review.

In summary, there is now a consensus regarding appropriate symptom control measures for patients lacking capacity in the last few days of life, and guidance on those measures is presented in the nationally recommended (and audited[9]) LCP. The areas where significant ethical controversy remains are: the use of medications to reduce respiratory secretions in unconscious patients; the issue of whether or not to commence or continue artificial hydration in the last few days of life; and occasionally the issue of sedation for distressed and agitated patients. Further evidence and discussion of the first two issues may well resolve the remaining clinical and ethical uncertainties. The third issue, sometimes called 'terminal sedation', we discuss as a separate topic in Chapter 6.

5.3.ii Moral problems when the patient is not imminently dying

When patients are believed to be in the last weeks or months of life due to identified conditions, and are not (so far as can be clinically ascertained) imminently dying, difficult ethical issues regarding symptom control can arise. There are three main reasons for this. The first is that interventions to alleviate symptoms more often entail practical procedures which, alongside potential to relieve suffering, are associated with harms and burdens, and some risks. Since these patients are not imminently dying, any harms and burdens resulting from symptom control measures may continue for a significant period. If the intervention is associated with a risk of death (as an adverse outcome) then life may be significantly shortened. The second reason is that such interventions may also alter the mode of death, as in the case of the examples listed in the discussion in Section 5.2 on issues arising where the patient has capacity.

The third reason is that the patient without capacity is not able to weigh up the benefits, harms and risks of the proposed intervention against his own priorities, make a choice, and give or withhold consent.

At the outset we must stress that a patient must not be assumed to lack capacity for a particular decision on the basis of appearance or a diagnosis such as dementia, learning disability, or mental illness; if there is any reason to doubt capacity it must be formally assessed. Patients must be given all appropriate and practicable assistance to make their own decisions before a judgement is made that they lack capacity. If it is then concluded that the patient does lack capacity, the decision-making process outlined in Section 2.5. is followed. But reaching a judgement about the patient's best interests may still be difficult. A fictional but realistic clinical scenario illustrates the difficulties.

An elderly lady, who had previously been living independently, was found to have bowel cancer after investigations for abdominal pain. Investigations including CT scans did not reveal any metastatic disease and so resection of the primary tumour was discussed at a bowel cancer multidisciplinary team meeting (participants included surgeons, radiologists and physicians). It was noted that she had quite severe ischaemic heart disease, and that consequently there was a significant risk that she might not survive the major surgery of a bowel resection or that she might suffer some other vascular adverse incident such as a myocardial infarction or cerebrovascular accident (stroke). The team decided that although she had some symptoms and signs of early intestinal obstruction, surgery was not appropriate and she should instead receive palliative care. It was explained to her that she had been found to have cancer, that surgery was too risky, and that medical treatment would be used to combat symptoms. Unfortunately, abdominal pain persisted and antispasmodics precipitated episodes of obstruction. The patient was not able to retain the information given to her, and continued to worry about her inability to eat, especially high fibre foods, which she believed were essential for her wellbeing. The physicians caring for her asked the surgeons to reconsider surgery to create a defunctioning colostomy to alleviate her symptoms and associated psychological distress. The patient was shown to have cognitive and memory impairment and assessment revealed that she lacked capacity for the complex decision regarding palliative surgery to create a defunctioning colostomy.

The decision in this case is complicated by factors such as the cardiovascular risks of even palliative surgery, the finding (after multiple explanations and demonstrations) that it was unlikely that she would be able to manage her own colostomy and so would require permanent residential care, and the fact that if her obstruction were relieved she might live to develop pelvic pain and other symptoms due to enlargement of the primary tumour mass.

Scenarios such as this are likely to become common as people live well into old age and develop dementia of varying degrees; one in four patients over the age of 80 years will have increasing dementia, alone or coexisting with other conditions.[10] Whereas it is possible for them to express their wishes, feelings and views about what matters to them, they may lack capacity for the complex decision which has to be made. Sometimes the interests of the patient with cognitive or memory impairment will best be served by trying an intervention (such as a syringe driver or blood transfusion), but then monitoring the effects and discontinuing the intervention if it proves excessively burdensome.

A clinical scenario which has recently caused controversy illustrates some lack of understanding about the basis for decisions regarding symptom control for demented patients. Dementia is acknowledged to be a terminal illness and patients with severe dementia would reasonably be described as requiring end of life care. Patients with dementia can suffer from agitation which is very distressing for them. Antipsychotic medications may reduce agitation and distress. A large epidemiological study published in 2008 appeared to demonstrate a significantly increased risk of stroke in patients with dementia who were being treated with antipsychotic drugs. The authors concluded that 'As the background risk of stroke in elderly patients is relatively high, we reaffirm that the risks associated with antipsychotic drug use in patients with dementia generally outweigh the potential benefits, and use of antipsychotic drugs in these patients should be avoided whenever possible.'[11] What is surprising is the conclusion that an increased risk of stroke should be taken to 'generally outweigh' the benefits of relief of agitation in patients who already have a terminal illness. Not surprisingly, this flawed conclusion was identified and criticized in a subsequent letter by a general practitioner. He eloquently describes the error of judgement as follows:

> Medicine once served to make patients better, alleviating symptoms and healing disease. Now it seems to have degenerated into a risk reducing, patient stratifying, life years adding bioscience disregarding the individual patient's needs. To deny a patient good treatment for disturbing and harassing complaints because of worries about possible side effects is unethical. Nobody would question prescribing morphine for terminal analgesia. Patients at the end of their life with dementia related behavioural problems should be able to expect proper treatment. To withhold this treatment for spurious and debatable reasons is 'madicine'.[12]

The guiding ethical principal in such cases must be treatment selection on the basis of the individual patient's best interests, which must depend in large part on the balance of benefit to harm and risk in that patient's case. The authors of the study had clearly not grasped this most basic principle, and the forthright criticism they received from the general practitioner is understandable and, in our view, justified!

John O'Brien, a professor of old age psychiatry, stated in a *BMJ* editorial, 'Prescriptions of antipsychotics should be carefully targeted, time limited, and reserved for severe and distressing symptoms after careful assessment of risk and benefit. This is not easy. How, for example, can we weigh up a small but real increased risk of stroke compared with the possible benefit of remaining in a less restricted environment (for example, at home)? These complex decisions have to involve the patient, where possible, together with the family and carers'.[13] In the context of end of life care, the benefit of being less distressed and possibly at home will surely often outweigh the small increased risk of stroke.

The Mental Capacity Act 2005 decision-making process for patients who lack capacity (see Section 2.5) does appear an ethically acceptable process for resolving such issues. It does require professional time and careful thought, discussion with the patient to listen to their views and ascertain sources of distress, and consultation within the health care team and with family and friends of the patient if available. It also requires willingness to review previous decisions if there are changes in the patient's condition and symptoms. Although it can be difficult, this decision-making responsibility is part of the professional role in end of life care, and it is a matter of ethical importance that it is carried out conscientiously.

5.4 **Conclusions**

1) Professionals are responsible for selecting symptom control treatment options so as to promote the patient's best interests; the balance of benefit relative to harm and risk determines the options which should be offered to patients with capacity, or considered for those lacking capacity.

2) Professionals ought to inform patients with capacity about possible serious adverse outcomes of symptom control interventions. In respect of less serious side-effects and risks, professionals must make clinical judgements about how much information should be given, since patients vary in their desire to receive it.

3) Decisions are made on behalf of patients who lack capacity on the basis of their best interests, taking into account the balance of benefit to harm and risk and what can be known of the patient's preferences and priorities. Consensus guidance is helpful in achieving comfort in the last few days of life.

References

1. General Medical Council (2008). *Consent: patients and doctors making decisions together.* GMC, London, para. 9.
2. GMC, op. cit. (ref. 1), para. 32.
3. GMC, op. cit. (ref. 1), para. 44.
4. GMC, op. cit. (ref. 1), p. 54.
5. Innes S, Payne S (2009). Advanced cancer patients' prognostic information preferences: a review. *Palliative Medicine* **23**:29–39.
6. Ellershaw JE, Wilkinson S (2003). *Care of the dying: a pathway to excellence.* Oxford University Press, Oxford.
7. Good P, Cavenagh J, Mather M, Ravenscroft P (2008). Medically assisted hydration for adult palliative care patients. *Cochrane Database of Systematic Reviews* 2008(2):CD006273.
8. Campbell C, Partridge R (2007). *Artificial nutrition and hydration: guidance in end of life care for adults.* National Council for Palliative Care, London.
9. Marie Curie Palliative Care Institute (2007). *National care of the dying audit—hospitals. Generic report 2006/7.* Marie Curie Institute, Liverpool. Available at http://www.mcpcil. org.uk (accessed 12.01.09).
10. Armitage M, Mungall I (2007). Palliative care services: meeting the needs of patients. *Clinical Medicine* **7**:436–8.
11. Douglas IJ, Smeeth L (2008). Exposure to antipsychotics and risk of stroke: self controlled case series study. *BMJ* **337**:a1227.
12. Conradi P (2008). Madness of modern medicine. *BMJ* **337**:a1670.
13. O'Brien J (2008). Antipsychotics for people with dementia. *BMJ* **337**:a602.

6

Choice and best interests: sedation to relieve otherwise intractable symptoms (terminal sedation)

We are discussing the problems of sedation under a separate heading for two reasons. First, this aspect of end of life care is currently the subject of much professional discussion and there are sufficient ethical issues arising from it to merit analysis as a separate topic. Second, the topic does not fit neatly into categories of patients with and without capacity because administering sedation to a patient with capacity can reduce alertness to the point that the patient then loses capacity; decisions about further sedation then have to be based on the patient's best interests.

There is considerable consensus on this topic and therefore we have included it in Part I of this book. In the UK, nationwide adoption of the Liverpool Care Pathway for the Care of the Dying (LCP) guidance on sedation in the last days of life is evidence of this consensus.[1] But there is also controversy about the ethical acceptability of the use of sedation in some clinical circumstances. To provide clarity our discussion will cover the following areas under subheadings: identifying the moral problems; what makes the analysis difficult; clinical circumstances where there is consensus; clinical circumstances which are controversial; solution via doctrine of double effect; solution via professional guidelines.

6.1 Identifying the problems

At the outset we can identify the moral problems which may be associated with sedation in end of life care:

1) the possibility that the sedation may hasten or even cause death;

2) the significant other harms and risks of sedation;

3) the moral relevance (or not) of the interests of others, including relatives and staff;

4) the separate issue of whether artificial hydration (and possibly nutrition) is appropriate during sedation.

We will discuss these problems in Sections 6.3 and 6.4 but we must first clear the ground by disposing of some serious impediments to clear discussion.

6.2 **What makes the analysis difficult**

There are three serious impediments to clear discussion of the ethical problems listed in Section 6.1. We shall discuss these in turn.

6.2.i **Lack of a clear definition of 'terminal sedation'**

Since there is a lack of clear definition of the concept of 'terminal sedation', so there is a notable lack of shared understanding of what practices are under discussion. We shall mention the various practices with which the term has been associated.

The term 'terminal sedation' appears in papers from the USA and Canada in 1996 and has been in use since.[2,3] But there is an ethically important ambiguity about the adjective 'terminal'. Whereas it can be interpreted as indicating sedation given to those imminently dying, it can also be taken to imply that the sedation was given with the intention of hastening or causing death, as it tends to be conflated with the concept of 'termination' and intention to 'terminate'. So the term is open to interpretation as some form of deliberately causing the end of life, which is not the meaning which most authors would intend. On the other hand, supporters of the legalisation of euthanasia might well prefer this term, on the basis that if terminal sedation (with connotations of intention to terminate life) is legally permitted, so should euthanasia be.

Lack of clarity about the meaning of 'terminal sedation' was evident and by 1998, following a postal survey of palliative care experts in eight countries, it was recommended that the term 'terminal sedation' be abandoned in favour of the descriptive phrase 'sedation for intractable distress in the dying.'[4] This suggestion might have been helpful but it was not generally adopted.

The term 'continuous deep sedation' has been used recently by writers from The Netherlands who use it to refer to continuously and deeply sedating a patient or keeping the patient in coma until death.[5] This term could be taken to mean treatment intended only to relieve intractable suffering in the last few days of life. But it could also mean maintaining a patient who was not imminently dying in a state of deep sedation until death occurred, either with the intention of alleviating suffering or with the intention of hastening or causing death. Unfortunately, this term was then misused by a British psychiatrist in relation to the use of benzodiazepines as recommended in the LCP.[6] The LCP recommends the carefully titrated use of midazolam, beginning with intermittent administration as needed to alleviate distress, and progressing to continuous administration only if frequent doses are required. The recommendations of the LCP do not equate to the concept of continuous deep sedation as described by the Dutch authors. So this term is unfortunately also ambiguous, and has in addition proved open to what is obviously misuse.

Other writers have preferred the term 'palliative sedation'. The problem with the adjective 'palliative' is that it also has a range of meanings. It can mean the opposite of 'curative', or it might refer to the context of palliative care, or it could refer to any form of sedation to palliate symptoms, even including night sedation in end of life care. In 2007 an international panel of 'palliative care experts' reviewed the evidence on this topic and produced recommendations for clinical practice, which are helpful. They use the term 'palliative sedation therapy', avoiding the word 'terminal' for the reasons we outlined above. They propose the following definition, including explanation of the term 'refractory':

> Palliative sedation therapy is the use of specific sedative medications to relieve intolerable suffering from refractory symptoms by a reduction in patient consciousness.... Refractory symptoms are symptoms for which all possible treatment has failed, or it is estimated that no methods are available for palliation within the time frame and the risk–benefit ratio that the patient can tolerate.[7]

This definition does indicate that the intention is to relieve severe and intractable (refractory) symptoms, and also that the means is intentional reduction of consciousness. The word 'palliative' implies that the patient is terminally ill, but it does not imply that the patient is imminently dying, so this definition could still apply to a range of clinical circumstances.

Lack of a clear and universally adopted definition makes it impossible to gain information about the use of sedation at the end of life. For example, on the basis of limited data from the USA it has been that suggested that the practice of terminal sedation 'accounts for 0–44% of deaths, depending on definitions and programmes'.[8] Part of the reason for this huge variation in the apparent use of sedation is thus attributed to marked variations in what counts as terminal sedation.

Readers will be relieved to hear that we shall not attempt to coin yet another term. Instead, we shall focus on the range of activities to which the existing terms might refer, analysing ethical acceptability for the use of sedation in each context. We shall be discussing sedation to achieve relief of otherwise intractable symptoms in the context of end of life care. We shall not be referring to the ethically unproblematic use of night sedation, or to the use of anxiolytics to calm a patient but not to reduce alertness.

6.2.ii Lack of clarity about the fundamental moral concepts of intention, outcome and causality in decision-making about sedation

Intention

Throughout the book we have stressed that health care professionals must intend only the benefits of achieving the three central aims of health care, namely relief of suffering, prolongation of life and restoration or maintenance of function. In Section 3.1 we discussed the important distinction between intending and foreseeing an outcome. Throughout our discussions we have stressed the importance of weighing up the intended benefit of an intervention against the foreseen harms and risks. In Section 3.3, we noted that health care professionals in the great majority of countries are prohibited from intentionally causing the deaths of their patients, in order to maintain societal prohibitions against killing which protect all members of those societies.

We have also noted the importance of being honest and open with ourselves and others regarding our intentions, even though this can be difficult, and we acknowledge that there can be a subliminal element to intention. The ensuing discussion will be based on the premise that in administering sedation to alleviate suffering the professional is under an ethical obligation not to intend to cause or hasten death. We shall mention in passing the rare exception to this which occurs in The Netherlands where euthanasia is legalized and so physicians are legally permitted to intend to cause (and then actually to cause) the patient's death.

Outcome

The outcome, or consequence, of a decision or action is clearly of moral impor-tance (although of course it is not the only factor which is important). The intended outcome of sedation is alleviation of distress. Unfortunately adverse outcomes can arise, such as increasing distress from being in a 'twilight' state with some disorientation and perhaps inability to communicate. The adverse outcome which causes most concern is any potential to hasten or cause death.

Causation

Causation is of great importance when, whilst under the effects of sedation, the patient dies. The morally important issue here is what was the cause of death. Causation is a complex concept, but in health care and health care law a simple approach is required. If the patient dies while sedated it is very important to ask the 'But for' question; in other words, 'But for the sedation would the patient have died?' This helps to elucidate what the patient has actually died of, or putting it another way, what caused death.

6.2.iii **Artificial hydration**

The third impediment to analysis is the issue of whether artificial hydration (and sometimes nutrition) is commenced or continued during sedation. We consider that this issue should be addressed as a separate decision, so that artificial hydration is considered on its own merit in relation to symptom control. In this we agree with the authors of the recommendations for clinical practice and other experienced clinicians.[9,10] But there is a complication in that it has been suggested that sedation maintained for a prolonged period in a patient who refuses concurrent artificial hydration could be used as a way to intentionally hasten death.[11] We shall discuss this controversial combination of prolonged sedation and refusal of hydration in our section on controversial clinical circumstances.

6.3 **Clinical circumstances where there is consensus**

Having cleared the ground of impediments to clear discussion, we shall now consider the substantive ethical issues. We can consider first the situation where *a patient has capacity* for the decision about sedation, is imminently dying but has intractable physical symptoms, and requests sedation.

An example would be a patient very distressed by dyspnoea due to tracheal obstruction by tumour, with audible stridor and impending critical loss of airway. If tracheostomy were not practicable or clinically appropriate, or if the patient had declined it, the patient might request sedation in order to be less aware of, and less distressed by, the increasing inability to breathe. We can assume that opiates and oxygen had already been used without relief of distress. The patient will die because of the loss of an adequate airway. There is a possibility that death might be hastened very slightly if sedation causes a decrease in respiratory drive, but this is unlikely. Death will occur with or without the sedation. The intended benefit of alleviation of severe and otherwise intractable distress greatly outweighs the small risk of hastening death, and the patient consents to the treatment having understood the clinical situation. Rapid titration of sedation would be used so as to give what is required while avoiding overdose. The sedation is thus both adequate and proportionate to the situation. Sedation sufficient to relieve distress is justifiable, even if it is necessary to reduce awareness and consciousness in order to obtain that relief. Indeed it would be very difficult, if not impossible, to justify refusing to provide sedation adequate to relieve distress in this situation.

Similar situations will occasionally arise in respect of severe and intractable psychological distress in an imminently dying patient who retains capacity for this decision. In this situation, sedation to produce a marked anxiolytic effect but without rendering the patient unresponsive or unconscious may well be effective. Such a treatment is an adequate and proportionate response to the situation and is justifiable if it accords with the patient's wishes. If the patient is panic-stricken and reassurance has not been effective, then it may be necessary to use larger doses to diminish consciousness, but this too would be a proportionate response and would be justifiable.

We shall now consider the common situation where a patient who is imminently dying becomes confused or semi-conscious as a result of the underlying illness and so *lacks capacity*. In that situation decisions about alleviating distress manifested by agitation and restlessness are taken on the basis of the patient's best interests (having treated any remediable causes of physical discomfort). The process of making decisions for patients who lack capacity was described in Section 2.5. Guidelines regarding medication, such as the LCP, may be followed.[12] Within the UK there is a consensus that the recommendations of this pathway are ethically appropriate and represent good clinical practice.

The LCP recommends initially using small doses of midazolam subcutaneously on an 'as needed' basis, with dose titration to achieve relief of distress. A continuous infusion of this drug is recommended if, at review after 24 hours, three or more doses have been required. The use of this regimen to alleviate distress when death is believed to be imminent (as is the case when the LCP is followed) is not controversial. Withholding such symptom control would be highly controversial and likely to be judged unethical.

Moreover, there is evidence that sedation to alleviate distress in the last days of life does not shorten life. So there appears to be no evidence base for the concern that the moral problem of hastening death arises in this situation.[13]

We shall now mention two situations which arise where the patient is not imminently dying and where sedation is not contentious.

The first is a situation in which sedation is justifiable for a patient who lacks capacity, but professionals sometimes become confused about whether it is ethical and lawful to give it. Patients who are not imminently dying but who are confused and disoriented can become very agitated and distressed, and sometimes aggressive and paranoid. This scenario sometimes occurs if the patient has pre-existing cognitive impairment. If reassurance and the presence of loved ones (if available) fail, antipsychotic medication is tried. If this fails then sedation to alleviate distress may be judged to be in the patient's best interests. The practical problem is that the patient may refuse to take any medication. In this situation, assuming that it is in the patient's best interests to receive antipsychotic drugs and possibly sedation, it is ethically justifiable (and in the UK lawful) to give the medication covertly, perhaps by putting it into a drink. This is less traumatic to the patient than an injection. Covert medication in this case is not unethical because the patient lacks capacity for the decision so is not, in fact, 'refusing' the medication in a moral and legal sense.

The second situation in which the patient is not imminently dying and sedation is not contentious arises when a patient with capacity has severe emotional distress. Sometimes patients remain psychologically distressed and unable to obtain relief from their worries and fears while awake. They can be offered intermittent sedation, timed to ensure they have a rest period during the day but are awake when visitors come and to take whatever food and fluids they want. Overnight sedation with continuous subcutaneous midazolam for 12 hours or less is often helpful to them. These measures are not controversial because the sedation is not continuous and so the benefits clearly outweigh the harms and risks and the patient is involved in the discussion and gives consent.

We have given these 'consensus' examples to illustrate the principle that the justification for the sedation is the balance of benefit to harm and risk in the individual case, plus the patients' consent when they have capacity, or their best interests when they lack capacity. In the above examples the sedation is not causing death, and it is also very unlikely that it is hastening death—death occurs as a result of the underlying illness. The international panel who produced recommendations for clinical practice were similarly describing situations where the use of sedation would not be contentious, as the intent is to alleviate suffering for which it is a proportionate response, it does not shorten life, and it raises 'no distinct ethical problem'.[14]

6.4 Clinical circumstances which are controversial

In this section we shall finally return to the ethical problems we listed at the start in Section 6.1.

In those situations in end of life care where significant sedation is controversial, the basis of the controversy is the identification of one or more of the moral problems listed in Section 6.1. So the moral problem might be the risk that sedation might hasten (or in extreme cases cause) death, that other harms and risks of sedation might outweigh the benefits, that the decision has been made on the basis of the interests of others and not those of the patient, and where poor fluid intake during prolonged sedation increases the risk that death may be hastened or caused. We shall discuss these moral problems in turn.

The first problem listed, *the risk of possibly hastening death* or even causing death, is the most obvious. The risk occurs if the patient is sedated continuously and is *not imminently dying*, and so immobility may predispose to chest infections, and fluid intake may fall below that required to sustain life. So continuous sedation to the point where the patient is semi-conscious or unconscious would, if prolonged, entail a risk of hastening death, or if very prolonged could conceivably cause death.

The amount of time by which life is shortened might be very difficult to estimate. This is because it can be very difficult to estimate the length of remaining life in some terminal illnesses; such prognostication is more difficult when the clinical signs of imminent death are not present. In chronic non-malignant conditions such as severe chronic obstructive pulmonary disease with exacerbations, and in heart failure, the patient's condition may deteriorate suddenly and unpredictably, making it very difficult to estimate prognosis. So whereas continuous sedation to a semi-conscious or uncon-scious state for a prolonged period would clearly entail a risk of hastening death, the degree to which life was in fact shortened would be almost impos-sible to judge. Nevertheless, it does seem morally more problematic to hasten death by several weeks than by one week, so the amount of time by which life may be shortened is morally relevant.

Clive Seale, a social scientist, studied end of life decisions by UK doctors and compared them with data from other countries. He found that UK doctors were less likely than doctors in other countries to state that they shortened life by more than one week but less than one month. He also found that UK doctors were more likely to state that life was shortened by less than one week than doctors in Australia and in countries which permit assisted suicide and euthanasia. He concluded that UK doctors are cautious about actions that significantly shorten life. In contrast, he found that in all countries actions which shortened life by an estimated time of more than one month were rare, and all the cases so described from the UK were actually decisions to withhold or withdraw a life-prolonging treatment.[15] A study of Canadian physicians and pharmacists working in palliative care centres also showed that the longer the patient's prognosis, the less the participants favoured sedation to alleviate either physical or emotional distress.[16] The international panel recommended that if sedation is continuous and deep then the disease should be advanced and irreversible with death expected within 'hours to days'.[17] Thus research suggests that it is generally considered more morally problematic to shorten life by more than one week, and very problematic to shorten it by more than one month.

A second factor to consider in the case of prolonged sedation with reduced consciousness, where the patient is not imminently dying, is the *inescapable uncertainty about the cause of death*. If the sedation is deep and prolonged and fluid intake is nil, then the sedation may have caused death. On the other hand, given that the context is end of life care and the patient is already very ill and expected to die in the near future, death might well have resulted from the underlying illness. As we noted early in our discussion, the cause of death is a morally relevant factor.

A third, and very important, factor is *the intention of the health care staff* prescribing and administering the sedation. We have noted that there is a general prohibition against intending to cause the patient's death (except in those very few jurisdictions in which euthanasia is lawful). We would argue (as did the international panel[18]) that there are very good, if not overwhelming, grounds for maintaining such prohibition, and that there are also grounds for ensuring that it clearly applies to health care professionals to whom the welfare of very vulnerable people is entrusted. This leads us to the conclusion that sedation with intent to cause or hasten death is not ethically acceptable.

A highly controversial practice was discussed by Quill and Byock in 2000.[19] They reported that a small percentage of terminally ill patients have intractable suffering and that some of these patients request that 'death be hastened'. They suggested 'terminal sedation' plus 'voluntary refusal' of hydration and nutrition 'as potential last resorts to address the needs of such patients'. They commented that this practice can 'substantially increase patients' choices.' This proposal is ethically highly problematic, as the following analysis reveals. We would judge it to be ethically unacceptable in patients who are not imminently dying; we therefore conclude that it should not be made available as a 'choice' for patients.

The patient is requesting prolonged sedation to semi-consciousness or unconsciousness, and at the same time is making what amounts to an advance refusal of hydration and nutrition when sedated by the health care staff. The proposal entails that the physician strives to maintain reduced consciousness, and consequently the patient is not able to reconsider the decision. The clear aim/intention of the proposal, as explained by these authors, is to hasten death. If the sedation were prolonged for a critical period, possibly in excess of one week, death due to the underlying illness would very probably be hastened. It is also possible that total lack of fluid intake for this period could, in itself, cause acute renal failure and death. So the intention is to hasten death, and the sedation combined with the patient's refusal of hydration is very likely to hasten death and may actually cause death.

The proposal is analogous to asking an anaesthetist to give a prolonged general anaesthetic to such a patient, and continue to keep the patient unconscious, without provision of fluids, until death occurred. In the proposal presented by Quill and Byock, assuming that the patient is not imminently dying, the physician's provision of prolonged and heavy sedation in the context of the patient's advance refusal of hydration has the moral features of euthanasia; the doctor's intention was to cause death, and the treatment given probably does cause death.

This is the conclusion reached by a group of authors from The Netherlands writing in 2008. They made the following distinction:

> When the patient's life expectancy is short [limit of one to two weeks mentioned] when sedation is started, continuous deep sedation presumably has no or only a limited effect on life shortening and is generally not considered to be the moral equivalent of euthanasia. When it is used for patients with a longer life expectancy with the intention to hasten the patient's death at his or her request, however, this practice should be regarded as the moral equivalent of euthanasia.[20]

We concur with this conclusion on the grounds that the intention is to hasten or possibly cause death, and the treatment is extremely likely to hasten or cause death, so intention and cause of death and outcome are the same as in euthanasia. We conclude that this practice is ethically not justifiable.

Whereas this is our view and likely to be a consensus view, since most countries prohibit euthanasia, the situation in The Netherlands appears to be different. In a study published in 2004, physician reports on sedation without hydration indicated that in 47% of such cases 'hastening death was partly the intention of the physician' and was 'the explicit intention' in 17% of cases. The authors concluded that 'Terminal sedation precedes a substantial number of deaths in The Netherlands. In about two-thirds of most recently reported cases, physicians indicated that in addition to alleviating symptoms, they intended to hasten death.'[21]

Apart from the moral problem of intentionally hastening or causing the patient's death, attempting to achieve prolonged sedation to lack of awareness in a patient not imminently dying entails the moral problem of risk of other harms. Assuming that sedation is not effected by a form of general anaesthetic, it may be quite difficult to sustain the level of diminished consciousness required to abolish awareness of unpleasant sensations, either mental or physical. So the patient might suffer 'twilight' periods of some awareness. The worst possibility would be a state of awareness with distress and possibly discomfort, but without adequate ability to signal distress. It is also possible that partial wakening could be associated with disorientation and distressing confusion. The practical clinical problems of ensuring that the patient is continuously and sufficiently sedated to avoid distress result in a real risk of harm to the patient.

The underlying premise of the above discussion was that the patient, prior to sedation, had capacity and requested prolonged sedation while making an advance refusal of fluids and food. If the patient at the outset lacked capacity and was not imminently dying, but professionals commenced and continued the prolonged sedation, then whether or not the sedation was morally justifiable would depend on the following factors: intention, causation of death, the extent to which life was shortened, and the potential of harms to the patient during the period of sedation. Consideration of all these factors would be necessary to judge whether such sedation was ethically justifiable in that particular case. In such a difficult (and probably rare) situation the doctrine of double effect, which we mention in Section 3.1, and will describe in detail below, can be used to judge whether the sedation is morally justifiable or not. Having resolved the issue of whether the sedation was morally justifiable, professionals would have to make the separate but linked judgement about whether or not artificial hydration should be provided. That judgement would be made on the basis of the patient's best interests.

In the discussion so far in this section we have analysed the moral problems of hastening or causing death and of risk of other harms where patients who are not imminently dying are continuously sedated. In the clinical situations we have described the decision has been made on the basis of the wishes or interests of the patient (see Section 6.1). We shall now discuss the major ethical problems of sedating a patient to pursue the interests of others. Any decision which is based on the interests of persons other than the patient is ethically problematic and inherently unlikely to be justifiable, and so ought to be controversial!

In the case of patients who are imminently dying, there is sometimes a conflict of interests between the patient and the relatives, between the dying patient and other patients, and between the patient and staff. We shall consider these in turn. In this discussion we are not implying that relatives or staff or indeed other patients are wicked or necessarily morally at fault, but we are realistic that they will have their own interests, and human beings are influenced by their own interests.

If an imminently dying patient still has capacity it is clear that whether or not sedation is given must depend only on the balance of benefit to harm and risk for the patient, plus the patient's consent or refusal. It would not be morally justifiable to sedate such a patient, against the patient's wishes, to further the interests of either relatives or staff. If the patient appears emotionally distressed despite efforts to resolve this, and the patient refuses sedation as a last resort, the relatives might well ask for the patient to be sedated. Their request is likely to be based on their view of the patient's interests as well as their own interests. It is very upsetting and even traumatic for relatives to sit by a dying loved one who is distressed. In this situation the staff may have similar feelings and motivation.

But it simply is not justifiable to impose the sedation on the patient with capacity who is refusing it. Nor should the sedation be given covertly (e.g. hidden in a drink).

If the imminently dying patient lacks capacity, the decision should be made on the basis of the patient's best interests. As we explained in Section 2.5, the best interests judgement includes what can be known of the patient's wishes and feelings, beliefs and values. Whether or not the patient should be sedated depends primarily on the balance of benefit to harm for the patient, but if there is clear evidence that the patient would have wanted the interests of relatives taken into consideration then it is legitimate to do so. However, there is a moral and legal limit to how far the interests of relatives should be taken into account on this basis.

For example, distressed relatives sometimes express the wish that 'it should all be over' and some even request that death be intentionally hastened, perhaps for their own sakes and perhaps because they believe it to be in the patient's interests. At other times relatives may find it distressing to sit with a patient who is aware and appears awake but is unable to communicate, and because of their distress they might ask that the patient be sedated so as to be 'asleep'. But the only morally acceptable course here is to treat the patient according to the patient's best interests. Even if professionals have grounds to believe that the patient would have taken the relatives' interests into account, that could not justify sedation which was not consistent with the best possible balance of benefit to harm and risk for the patient. It is clearly not acceptable to sedate a patient who is not distressed in order to comply with the wishes of relatives or to reduce their distress.

This conclusion may appear obvious, but professionals might still act in the interests of the relatives and contrary to those of the patient for two reasons. The first is that the philosophy of palliative care, which has been highly influential in end of life care, has always stressed the importance of care for the patient's family, and indeed it has included improvement of the quality of life of the family within the aims of palliative care. Professionals influenced by this philosophy might consider that they have a duty to further the interests of the relatives even when these interests conflict with those of the patient. For example, the international panel of palliative care experts recommended that staff should 'act creatively to meet the needs of the patient and their family', and suggested tailoring sedating interventions to the patient's and/or family's values.[22] The second reason is that in situations where all concerned are distressed it can be difficult for professionals to retain the ability to see the morally relevant issues clearly and weigh them up rationally. Although both of these reasons provide explanations, they are not justifications for compromising the interests of the patient in order to further those of the relatives.

It is clearly not acceptable to compromise the interests of the imminently dying patient for the sake of the interests of the staff. But it is important to distinguish between the interests of the staff and those of other patients to whom the staff do owe a duty of care (both morally and legally). When patients are being cared for in an institutional setting, either in a nursing home or hospital ward, it occasionally happens that a patient who is imminently dying is making sounds which are distressing to other patients. If the dying patient is groaning this is likely to be a sign of discomfort and appropriate treatment should of course be given. But if it is just a noise in the patient's throat during expiration, with no signs of distress, then staff may consider giving medications such as midazolam with the aim of alleviating the distress of other patients. Whether or not this is justifiable depends on the balance of benefit to harm for the dying patient—it can perhaps be justified if there is no harm or risk to the dying patient, and if alternative measures to alleviate the distress of other patients (e.g. explanation and reassurance) have failed.

We have discussed the moral problems of conflicts of interest where the patient is imminently dying. Where the patient is not imminently dying it appears impossible to justify prolonged and continuous sedation, which is not in the interests of the patient, for the sake of benefit to relatives, staff or other patients. Decisions about sedation for such patients should be taken on the basis of their own interests (and their consent or refusal if they have capacity). The only exception is where aggressive behaviour is significantly compromising the safety and comfort of other patients, or the safety of staff. In that situation intermittent sedation, or mild sedation, may well be justifiable. By contrast, continuous and prolonged sedation to a state of diminished consciousness would not be.

Finally, we must consider the separate but linked decision regarding artificial hydration, and occasionally nutrition via nasogastric or percutaneous endoscopic gastrostomy tube (Section 6.1). It is important that this decision is not somehow conflated with that regarding sedation. The decision about artificial hydration and nutrition must be taken on the basis of the balance of benefit to harm and risk for that particular treatment in the circumstances, plus consideration of the patient's priorities as we noted in 6.2.iii. The decision-making processes described in Chapter 2 should be followed. The international panel noted that artificial hydration may be indicated if sedation is intended to be transient, or is considered for a patient with life expectancy of more than 1 week.[23] The only exception (which we have already discussed) is where a patient who is not imminently dying has made a legally binding advance refusal of artificial hydration and then requests prolonged and continuous sedation, stipulating that the advance refusal of hydration should apply during the sedation. In this case the professional's decision about sedation is rightly influenced by the patient's advance refusal.

From this lengthy discussion it is evident that decision-making regarding sedation towards the end of life is complex, and professionals will need some guidance in decision-making. There are two solutions which could provide such guidance. The first is the correct application of the doctrine of double effect, and the second is the production of explicit professional guidance on what is ethically (and legally) acceptable and what is not.

6.5 Solution to the problems via the doctrine of double effect

This doctrine is mentioned in Section 3.1 where we noted that it may be invoked to judge whether an act with a foreseen bad effect (of possibly shortening life) is justifiable. We describe and discuss the doctrine in more detail in the online Appendix at Section A10.3.

We must first note that the doctrine does not apply where sedation is appropriately used in the last days of life (as in the LCP) because sedation so used does not shorten life, as evidenced by multiple retrospective studies (cited by the international panel). Since there is no 'bad effect' requiring justification, the doctrine of double effect is not relevant. We do not agree, however, with those who suggest that an effect of hastening death at the end of a terminal illness should not be regarded as an untoward or bad effect;[24] in end of life care such an argument could lead to weakening of the prohibition against intending to cause or hasten death, or to the provision of highly risky treatment on the basis that hastening death was not an adverse effect. It must also be remembered that the doctrine cannot justify euthanasia (see online Appendix).

If we now consider continuous and prolonged sedation in patients not imminently dying, we can note that such treatment is very unlikely to be justifiable according to the four conditions of the doctrine. If the intention of such sedation is to cause or hasten the patient's death, the second condition is not met because the bad effect is intended. If life is significantly shortened or if it is likely that the sedation causes death, then the fourth condition of proportionality is likely not to be met, because the bad effect is likely to outweigh the good effect. The doctrine has a theoretical potential to differentiate between justifiable and unjustifiable use of sedation in those cases where it has a possible foreseen effect of shortening life.

However, we noted in Section 3.1 and the online Appendix that whereas the doctrine could theoretically be used to judge whether or not a particular symptom control intervention is morally justifiable, its use in the clinical setting is problematic and may not be desirable. It is also not necessary in the great majority of cases where the relative balance of benefit to harm and risk is sufficient to justify sedation. But advocates of the doctrine might wish to use its four conditions to analyse cases where sedation is likely to significantly hasten or cause death, because such decisions are recognized as being very difficult and controversial. There is, however, an alternative solution which we shall now mention.

6.6 Solution via professional guidelines

Health care staff are increasingly familiar with the use of protocols and guidelines and it may be possible to draw up consensus guidance on the use of continuous sedation in end of life care. Such guidance would indicate what ought to be done in different sorts of clinical situation. Since what is actually being done is not necessarily what ought to be done, it is not possible or appropriate to formulate guidance on what ought to be done merely on the basis of surveys reporting current clinical practice.

Following an extensive literature review, the expert international panel produced recommendations designed to direct clinical practice; they recommended that to warrant continuous and deep sedation at the end of life, the patient's condition should be irreversible and advanced, with death expected within hours to days.[25] They gave detailed guidance on the decision-making process and on titration of sedation so as to give only what is required to alleviate distress, and noting that continuous and deep or sudden sedation is justified only in exceptional circumstances. Such guidance might be a more practicable solution to the clinical ethical problems of sedation to achieve relief of otherwise intractable symptoms in end of life care.

Guidance on sedation at the end of life is necessary to prevent its misuse in situations where adequate attempts have not been made to alleviate physical and mental distress, either because of failure to seek appropriate expert advice or because of lack of resources. Such misuse is obviously ethically unacceptable when expertise and resources are accessible. This point was made by authors from the disciplines of primary care, specialist palliative care, and anaesthetics who noted in a *BMJ* editorial that:

> there is a legitimate concern that sedation should not become a substitute for meticulous assessment and intensive treatment of physical symptoms and psychological or spiritual distress. Specialist palliative care teams regularly help patients with

previously intractable pain, delirium, anxiety, or dyspnoea become more comfortable. Palliative care is personalised and costly, while sedation is a relatively inexpensive, one size fits all treatment.[26]

Guidance could also helpfully stress that professionals, patients, and relatives must understand that treatment decisions made at a particular time and in particular circumstances are valid only at that time and in those circumstances. Treatment decisions need to be reviewed regularly, at least as often as significant changes in the patient's condition or wishes occur, or if other circumstances affecting their care change. No treatment decision is written in tablets of stone.

Moreover, since there are so many uncertainties in the factors considered when end of life care decisions are made, many decisions will turn out with hindsight not to have given the optimum result, and the treatments will need to be changed or modified.

6.7 Anticipating loss of capacity

In end of life care, professionals can often foresee likely events in the course of the illness which might cause the patient to lose capacity for decisions which may have to be made. When possible, and without causing distress or trauma to the patient, it is good practice to attempt to discuss with patients what treatment they would want if these events took place and they then lacked capacity to make their own choices between treatment options. Such discussions are now called advance care planning discussions, and any record made of the patient's preferences (with the patient's full agreement to the record) is called an advance statement.

For example, some patients want to remain as alert as possible so long as they have capacity, but they are also of the view that once they have lost capacity their priority would be comfort. Such patients might wish to inform their professional carers that in the event of loss of capacity they would prefer that their comfort was the highest priority, and that side-effects of sedation would be acceptable to them to achieve comfort.

When best interests judgements become necessary because of loss of capacity it is very helpful for professionals to have knowledge of the patient's previously expressed preferences. But it is of the utmost ethical importance that professionals understand and accept that advance care planning discussions are voluntary for patients; many patients will not want to try to foresee future illness scenarios, and it is easy to traumatize them by initiating or pursuing discussions about future events in order to make future decision-making easier.

We discussed the many contentious aspects of advance care planning in Chapter 7.

6.8 Conclusions

1. Sedation may be justifiable in order to alleviate otherwise intractable distress towards the end of life. But where there is a risk of hastening death or of other harms, the intended benefit must be proportionate to the foreseen harms and risks in order to justify the sedation. The doctrine of double effect is helpful in determining whether the sedation is ethically justifiable in a particular case, but in clinical practice professional guidelines may be more practicable.

2. Decisions must be frequently reviewed as patients' clinical circumstances change due to progressive disease, and there are many uncertainties in decision-making in end of life care.

References

1. Ellershaw JE, Wilkinson S (2003). *Care of the dying: a pathway to excellence*. Oxford University Press, Oxford.
2. Mount B (1996). Morphine drips, terminal sedation, and slow euthanasia: definitions and facts, not anecdotes. *Journal of Palliative Care* 12:21–30.
3. Rousseau P (1996). Terminal sedation in the care of dying patients. *Archives of Internal Medicine* 156:1785–6.
4. Chater S, Viola R, Paterson J, Jarvis V (1998). Sedation for intractable distress in the dying—a survey of experts. *Palliative Medicine* 12:255–69.
5. Rietjens J, van Delden J, Onwuteaka-Philipson B, Buiting H, van der Maas P, van der Heide A (2008). Continuous deep sedation for patients nearing death in the Netherlands: descriptive study. *BMJ* 336:810–3.
6. Treloar A (2008). Continuous deep sedation: Dutch research reflects problems with the Liverpool care pathway. *BMJ* 336:905.
7. De Graeff A, Dean M (2007). Palliative sedation therapy in the last weeks of life: a literature review and recommendations for standards. *Journal of Palliative Medicine* 10:67–85.
8. Quill TE (2007). Physician assisted deaths in vulnerable populations. *BMJ* 335:625–6.
9. De Graeff, Dean, op. cit. (ref. 7), p. 75.
10. Murray SA, Boyd K, Byock I (2008). Continuous deep sedation in patients nearing death. *BMJ* 336:781–2.
11. Quill TE, Byock IR (2000). Responding to terminal suffering: the role of terminal sedation and voluntary refusal of food and fluids. *Annals of Internal Medicine* 132:408–14.
12. Marie Curie Palliative Care Institute (2008). Liverpool Care Pathway for the Dying Patient (LCP). http://www.mcpcil.org.uk/liverpool_care_pathway
13. Sykes N, Thorns A (2003). Sedative use in the last week of life and the implications for end-of-life decision making. *Archives of Internal Medicine* 163:341–4.

14. De Graeff, Dean, op. cit. (ref. 7), pp. 76–7.

15. Seale C (2006). Characteristics of end-of-life decisions: survey of UK medical practitioners. *Palliative Medicine* **20**:653–9.

16. Blondeau D, Roy L, Dumont S, Godin G, Martineau I (2005). Physicians' and pharmacists' attitudes toward the use of sedation at the end of life: influence of prognosis and type of suffering. *Journal of Palliative Care* **21**:238–45.

17. De Graeff, Dean, op. cit. (ref. 7), p. 70.

18. De Graeff, Dean, op. cit. (ref. 7), p. 76.

19. Quill, Byock, op. cit. (ref. 11).

20. Rietjens *et al.*, op. cit. (ref. 5), p. 810.

21. Rietjens J, van der Heide A, Vrakking AM, Onwuteaka-Philipsen B, van der Maas P, van der Wal G (2004). Physician reports of terminal sedation without hydration or nutrition for patients nearing death in the Netherlands. *Annals of Internal Medicine* **141**:178–85.

22. De Graeff, Dean, op. cit. (ref. 7), pp. 72–3.

23. De Graeff, Dean, op. cit. (ref. 7), p. 75.

24. De Graeff, Dean, op. cit. (ref. 7), p. 77.

25. De Graeff, Dean, op. cit. (ref. 7), pp. 71–5.

26. Murray *et al.*, op. cit. (ref. 10), p. 781.

Conclusion to Part 1

In Part 1 we assumed that 'patient choice' referred to the choices which the doctor offered the patient, with information to enable the patient to choose (i.e. consent to or refuse) what was on offer. We argued that seen in this way patient choice leads to joint decision-making. Joint decision-making respects the integrity of both patient and doctor and results in an ethically beneficial partnership.

In Part 1 the best interests of patients were shown to be promoted by means of the traditional aims of medicine: to prolong life, to alleviate suffering, and to restore or maintain function. Our claim was that these remain the aims of end of life care, with the qualification that in pursuing the aims the priorities of care must alter: the possibilities for restoring function are limited, and whereas the prolongation of life remains an aim in end of life care it is often subordinated to the alleviation of suffering. For example, whereas within curative medicine a patient might be willing to tolerate a period of pain and suffering (say involving an operation) where there is a good chance of substantial recovery, within end of life care there is no such prospect. Hence, the emphasis is rightly on the alleviation of suffering, even (in rare circumstances) at the cost of shortening life a little. Nevertheless, sometimes it is possible to prolong life to a limited extent in end of life care, so the prolongation of life remains an aim.

To understand decision-making in end of life care adequately it is necessary to appreciate the importance of three distinctions: between intended and foreseen consequences; between acts and omissions; and between killing and letting die. The sedation of patients with otherwise intractable suffering is a controversial area in end of life care. Many of the problems derive from confusions about the meaning of 'terminal sedation'; we clarify this concept, discuss those clinical practices on which there is consensus and identify and discuss those which are controversial.

Our hope in Part 1 was to express the current consensus on decision-making in end of life care as far as it goes, in the context of patient choice and best interests, and in accordance with official guidance from professional bodies such as the General Medical Council and British Medical Association and with the current UK law.

Part 2

Controversies

In Part 2 we shall consider the many views to the effect that our Part 1 interpretations of both 'patient choice' and 'best interests' simply do not go far enough. Patient choice, it might be argued, should not be restricted to the choices which the doctor offers. The choices should be whatever is available to the consumer of healthcare. These consumer choices should extend, at least, to advance care planning (Chapter 7) and to the preferred place of care and death (Chapter 8). It is even arguable that if consumer choice is the central idea of health care provision it should extend to physician-assisted suicide or even to euthanasia (Chapter 9).

If we turn now to 'best interests' it might also be argued that whereas prolonging life, alleviating suffering, and improving function are certainly aspects of a patient's best interests, these interests are much wider and deeper, especially in end of life care. We shall therefore consider the view that the traditional 'best interests' of health care should be extended to include psychosocial and spiritual wellbeing (Chapter 10). Indeed, those approaching end of life ethics from a specialist palliative care point of view might wish to take the matter even further and argue that the interests of relatives as well those of the patient should be of concern to the practitioner (Chapter 10).

In a concluding chapter we shall try to pull together the strands in the book and provide an overview of the issues. In particular, we shall suggest criteria which an acceptable approach to end of life care should satisfy, and we shall leave it to the reader to decide how far the recent political, consumerist approach can meet the criteria.

Choice and advance care planning (ACP): definition, professional responsibilities

End of life care will often require treatment and care decisions, including those pertaining to life-prolonging treatment, to be made on behalf of patients who no longer have capacity to make such decisions for themselves. The great majority of those decisions will be made by health care professionals on the basis of the patient's best interests, a process which we explain in Section 2.5. It is helpful in making a best interests judgement if there is some record or knowledge of the patients' wishes and feelings, beliefs and values, when they had capacity, since these factors must be taken into account when making decisions once the patient has lost capacity.

Before we discuss the ethical issues arising in relation to such records or knowledge, we will explain the terminology which is used, as it has the potential to create real confusion.

In recent years it has become accepted practice for patients, while they have capacity, to record their wishes regarding treatment/care for a future time when they have lost capacity. That record might be a written statement, or a witnessed oral statement. The purpose of the statement is explicitly and only to influence decision-making if the patient loses capacity. It is called an 'advance statement' as it is written 'in advance of' future loss of capacity.

Advance statements are often referred to as 'living wills' and were previously called 'advance directives'. Since there is ambiguity regarding the precise meaning of both these terms they have now been superseded by the term 'advance statement'. The use of advance statements in health care has been relatively recent, and the first professional guidance was produced in the UK by the British Medical Association in the early 1990s.[1]

Patients sometimes want to make a refusal of certain treatments, to apply in the future when they have lost capacity, and perhaps to apply only in circumstances which they specify. This is an advance refusal of treatment and it is a subset of advance statements. Since refusal of treatment is the patient's decision, the Mental Capacity Act 2005 has referred to advance refusals of treatment as *advance decisions*.[2] Guidance on advance decisions is given in the Code of Practice which accompanies the Act.[3] This guidance explains the legal rules pertaining to their formulation and use in decision-making. In order to promote general understanding, such decisions by patients are often referred to as *advance decisions to refuse treatment* (ADRT).

When health care professionals are making decisions on behalf of a patient who lacks capacity, and they are presented with or find an advance statement of any sort (including an ADRT) which appears to be relevant to the decision in question, they must consider whether the statement is *valid*, and whether it is *applicable* in the current circumstances. The Mental Capacity Act Code of Practice gives guidance on the judgements of validity and applicability in relation to advance decisions (ADRTs) and the principles of this guidance should be applied by clinicians to advance statements which are not actually ADRTs. In other words, even though the great majority of advance statements are not ADRTs, professionals still have to make a judgement about whether they are valid and whether they are applicable to the current clinical circumstances in which a decision is required.

The philosophy of palliative care traditionally emphasized the importance of enhancing patients' ability to make choices and respecting those choices where possible. This idea, combined with the acceptance of advance statements in medical practice and common law, then evolved into a larger concept called *advance care planning* (ACP). This is the process of discussion between the patient (who has capacity) and a health care professional about the patient's preferences for future care in the event of loss of capacity. This discussion may, or may not, result in the patient making an advance statement depending on whether the patient wants a record of the discussion made.

This concept of ACP has been introduced into end of life care; in 2004 the National Institute for Clinical Excellence, in its guidance on supportive and palliative care for adults with cancer, recommended two documents to record ACP discussions.[4] Such recorded discussions constitute an advance statement, but they are often referred to as 'advance care plans'. Now the *End of life care strategy* (2008) also recommends ACP discussions and the formulation of advance statements.[5] The General Medical Council (GMC), in its 2008 guidance on consent, includes a section on ACP and recommends that the patient's views are recorded in a plan agreed with the patient—such a plan constitutes an advance statement.[6]

Such statements (or advance care plans) are seen as a way of continuing to exercise some form of choice even when capacity to make the relevant decision is lost, which is considered desirable for patients. Other potential advantages are: assisting professionals in making best interests judgements; making it easier for family members, who are consulted by professionals, to decide what they feel the patient would have wanted and what is in the patient's best interests; avoiding waste of resources where the statement indicates treatments that the patient would not want.

It must be noted that adults with capacity can make an advance decision to refuse treatment and it will be legally binding if it is found to be valid and applicable in the circumstances which later arise (when the patient has lost capacity) and if it meets the stipulations for formulation laid down in laws such as the Mental Capacity Act. Scotland has a separate Adults with Incapacity Act which is slightly different in detail but the issues are the same. (Law in other countries may be significantly different.) However, following case law, a request for treatment or care expressed in an advance statement is not legally binding in the UK (just as a patient with capacity cannot require health care professionals to provide treatment or care which those professionals judge is not clinically appropriate).[7] The legal background to this is summarized in two papers which are well referenced.[8,9] Thus a request for particular treatment or care expressed in an advance care plan document is not legally binding on health care professionals—this is sometimes not understood by professionals, patients or their relatives. However, the Mental Capacity Act stipulates that an advance statement/advance care plan must be taken into account when making best interests judgements on behalf of patients who have lost capacity.[10]

There is now a consensus in favour of the value of advance statements for those patients who wish to make them. Health care professionals and many members of the public have a broad understanding of what is involved. But there is much less agreement about the extent to which patients should be positively encouraged to undertake ACP discussions so as to think ahead about, and record, what they would or would not want in future situations where they had lost capacity to make the relevant decision. There is uncertainty about the overall balance of benefit to harm and risk for patients which might result from a policy of approaching patients to initiate ACP discussions. One of the national guidance documents on ACP notes that 'Further research on advance care planning (ACP) is necessary, both to evaluate the effect the ACP process itself may have on individuals, and to evaluate any interventions in care or treatment that may result from ACP.'[11] We therefore regard the introduction of ACP into end of life care as controversial, and so discuss it in Part 2 of this book.

In this chapter we shall outline the definition and main features of ACP, the professional responsibilities involved, common misunderstandings of it, and its evidence base. We shall conclude by examining the example of cardiopulmonary resuscitation (CPR) in the context of ACP. In Chapter 8 we shall concentrate on a particularly controversial aspect of it, which has been described as the 'preferred place of care and death' policy, a term we shall retain. Readers must decide for themselves whether the enthusiastic adoption of ACP in all its aspects will be good for patients and their families, whether it will achieve equity and cost-effectiveness in terms of resources, and also whether its use as a target or 'performance measure' for professionals will actually turn it into a stick with which politicians can beat the backs of professionals—with potential adverse consequences for patients and professionals alike.

7.1 **National guidance on ACP**

There are two authoritative national guidance documents on ACP. The first was produced by the End of Life Care Programme and was revised in 2008.[12] We have referred to this as the 'EoLCP' guidance. The second is evidence-based guidance from a group assembled by the British Geriatric Society and the Royal College of Physicians and published by the latter in 2009.[13] This group also had members from the Royal Colleges of General Practitioners, Psychiatrists, and Nursing, from the British Society of Rehabilitation Medicine and the National Council for Palliative Care, and from patients' groups such as Help the Aged and the Alzheimer's Society. We have referred to this guidance as the 'Joint' guidance in this chapter. A very short summary of it was published as a journal paper.[14]

National guidance on advance decisions to refuse treatment was produced in 2008.[15] It includes a suggested template to assist patients to write an ADRT so that it will be compliant with the requirements of the Mental Capacity Act.

The definition of ACP given in the EoLCP guidance is actually a description of many essential features:

> Advance care planning (ACP) is a voluntary process of discussion about future care between an individual and their care providers, irrespective of discipline. If the individual wishes, their family and friends may be included. It is recommended that with the individual's agreement this discussion is documented, regularly reviewed, and communicated to key persons involved in their care.

The definition goes on to state the topics which might be included in the discussion, in the following order: the individual's concerns, wishes, important values or personal goals for care, their understanding about their illness and prognosis, and their preferences and wishes for types of care or treatment that may be beneficial in the future and the availability of these.

The EoLCP guidance also makes clear at the outset the essential distinction between ACP and any other care planning:

> The difference between ACP and care planning more generally is that the process of ACP will usually take place in the context of an anticipated deterioration in the individual's condition in the future, with attendant loss of capacity to make decisions and/or ability to communicate wishes to others.

This last statement is an attempt to ensure that professionals understand that the ACP discussion, and any written plan which ensues from it, should be used only if and when the patient loses capacity. The guidance in its key principles also confirms that ACP requires the individual 'to have capacity to understand, discuss options available and agree to what is then planned'. So a patient who lacks this capacity cannot do ACP, for example if the patient already has dementia sufficiently severe to cause lack of capacity for the detailed discussion required. What is possible for such a patient is care planning more generally, but definitely not ACP.

The GMC guidance on consent also makes it clear that the purpose of ACP and recording of the patient's preferences is to make known the patient's wishes in the event of future loss of capacity.[16]

7.2 Who should have the discussion with the patient?

Both sets of national guidance stress that the professional having the discussion with the patient must have the relevant knowledge base, including the ethical and legal issues, plus the necessary communication skills. The Joint guidance group, based on evidence, recommended that 'The professional should have adequate knowledge about the disease, treatment and the particular individual to be able to give the patient all the information needed to express their preferences to make the plan.' They also recommended that professionals leading the discussion should, where necessary, have the support of another professional with the relevant specialist knowledge. Where training was concerned, they noted that staff required knowledge of the 'relevant disease process, prognosis and treatment options in order to undertake useful ACP discussions.' The EoLCP guidance includes as a key principle that 'health and social care staff should be aware of and give a realistic account of the support, services and choices available in the particular circumstances.' This will clearly involve knowledge about local community and secondary care services.

The ethical basis of these requirements is that patients must be given adequate information as a basis for making their own choices and expressing preferences. The ethical requirement to provide information for ACP is the same as that for contemporaneous decision-making in consent.

So the professional initiating and taking part in the discussion should be very knowledgeable and skilled, and should also be acquainted with the circumstances of the patient. Indeed, the range of knowledge and skills required is so large that it may only rarely be held by a single individual. This reality was recognized by members of the Joint guidance group (personal communication).

The Joint guidance group mention that the professional role could be carried out by 'a community matron or specialist nurse with the necessary expertise and knowledge base.' This is certainly possible, but community matrons have a wide remit, and specialist nurses, either in palliative care or disease specific, have limited availability and would require training. The obvious alternative, also requiring training, would be to use doctors either in the context of primary care or secondary care, probably in the outpatient setting. For example, the Joint guidance recommends that ACP should be considered in general practitioners' annual review of patients with long term conditions. But this is very expensive in terms of medical resources of manpower and money, especially as ACP is best conducted as an ongoing process, not as a single event. The Joint guidance 'top tips for successful ACP' state that discussions usually need to take place on more than one occasion and should not be completed on a single visit in most circumstances, and that they take time and effort and cannot be completed as a simple checklist exercise.

The ethical issues which arise are that the possibly scarce, and necessarily expensive, resources of manpower and money are likely to result in patients not having adequate opportunities for ACP with appropriately knowledgeable and skilled professionals. Instead patients may have ACP discussions with professionals who lack the essential elements of knowledge, skills or time. A further ethical issue is the opportunity cost to patients requiring interventions of immediate import, such as treatment now. They would compete for time against patients requiring recurring appointment slots long enough to undertake the ongoing discussions of ACP.

7.3 **When should ACP be instigated?**

The *End of life care strategy* boldly states, in a prominent box describing a recommended ACP document for patients called the *Preferred priorities for care* (PPC) document, that 'it is never too early to start a PPC plan'![17]

But can this claim be justified? Or can the reverse be shown, that it can be too early to start a PPC ACP document, or indeed inappropriate to start one at all?

The evidence-based guidance of the Joint guidance group notes that patients can demonstrate a range of responses to instigation of an ACP discussion; they noted that some patients have not wished and will not wish to consider ACP. Others will be willing to discuss some but not other aspects of care, and some would be prepared to make a verbal statement of their wishes but not to document them. Some are willing to document and review their wishes. Evidence also showed that 'Patients can exhibit several of these responses at once, and may oscillate between responses'. So the evidence demonstrated that for some patients ACP was not acceptable at a particular time, or perhaps never. It would seem that for some patients it can definitely be too early to start the PPC document!

Evidence was also found to the effect that ACP discussions at entry into a care home may cause additional upset at a time of transition, so the guidance advises that it should not be initiated until the patient is settled. Evidence also demonstrated that the instigation of ACP just after diagnosis of a terminal illness or during an inpatient stay following acute admission to hospital could cause undue distress (personal communication and published guidance). By contrast, the group noted that 'the majority of individuals are happy to discuss ACP in primary and outpatient care settings when their condition is stable, in anticipation of future ill-health'. But in the end of life care context the patient's condition is very often not stable, and the patient usually has current ill-health, rather than contemplating a future ill-health scenario. This may explain the finding that, in relation to participating in an ACP discussion, 'some patients with terminal disease or serious illness requiring hospitalization may not feel ready or able to do so'.

The Joint guidance recommends that 'ACP should be offered during routine clinical practice, but never forced upon an individual'. It also recommends that any approach to ACP should be straightforward and should allow the patient to close the topic down at any time, and that ACP discussions should not be continued if they are causing the patient excessive distress or anxiety. It therefore supports the *routine* instigation of ACP by professionals, albeit with readiness to discontinue the discussion.

But the EoLCP guidance is much more cautious. It stresses in its key principles that ACP is voluntary for patients, and that staff should instigate it *only if* they have made a professional judgement that it is likely to benefit the care of that individual. It also stresses, when considering timing, that ACP should not be initiated simply as part of routine record-keeping or care.

The explanation for this difference of views may lie in the differences between what people consider a theoretical ideal, and how they then feel in the reality of the situation. The Joint guidance group noted that 'most professionals and patients (>80%) agree that ACP discussions should take place around the time of diagnosis of a life-threatening illness'. Despite this comment on general views about ACP, their evidence demonstrated that, in reality, patients may not want ACP at this time. It appears that people are less enthusiastic about the concept of ACP when it is suggested for themselves after recent diagnosis of a terminal illness.

Although the EoLCP guidance suggests that professionals might instigate ACP following a new diagnosis of a life-limiting condition such as cancer or motor neurone disease, it is questionable whether that period immediately after learning the diagnosis, and probably prior to experiencing the effects of the illness and treatment, is really the right time to judge preferences for a future time when capacity is lost. What sounds like a good idea to profession-als, to patients not facing death, and to writers of the *End of life care strategy*, may not be a good idea for patients in the real context of end of life care. The same guidance suggests instigation of ACP if there have been multiple hospital admissions or a significant shift in treatment focus, but this contrasts with the evidence found by the Joint guidance group that instigation of ACP during acute admission to hospital could cause significant distress. So there exists considerable controversy regarding when/whether ACP should be instigated by professionals.

The ethically important point is that ACP is always voluntary for the patient.

Even more controversially, the EoLCP guidance suggests that professionals might instigate ACP (with people who are not necessarily ill) at the time of a life-changing event, citing the death of a spouse or close friend. But surely this period of intense sadness and adjustment to loss is hardly the best time to make judgements about what health care one might want or not want in the event of future loss of capacity!

Readers must judge for themselves from the evidence, and from their own professional and personal experience of people and life, whether it can, for the patient, be too early to instigate ACP and completion of the PPC document or similar. They might even conclude that for some patients ACP is never appropriate because of their attitude to their illness and to death.

7.4 **Information needed by patients for ACP regarding future treatment**

Patients considering treatment options in advance require information about those options in order to judge what they would and would not want at a future time when they have lost capacity. For each option patients will need to understand its potential benefits and its associated harms and risks, both in general but also with reference to their particular clinical situation. In other words, the information that they ought to be given is the same as they would require if giving contemporaneous consent (which we discuss in Sections 2.4.i and 4.4.i).

The Joint guidance recommends, in top tips for successful ACP discussions, that patients 'should be given sufficient information about their possible options and under what circumstances their plan would be activated. They need to understand what the consequences of their decision would be'. This advice is clearly ethically appropriate and should be followed, but it does mean giving patients a very substantial amount of information. Moreover, in the context of end of life care, this information is about possible illness scenarios and how treatment would alter them. It is very often about ways of dying (see Section 4.4.i).

Not only is much of this information unpleasant, but it may also turn out to be unnecessary; the discussion is about what may happen in the future, so must cover a range of possible or probable scenarios, some (or even all) of which will never happen. Yet in order to be adequately informed for ACP, patients must be given this substantial amount of (potentially) unpleasant information, which many will find distressing. Such distress can be construed as a harm. Furthermore, for the scenarios discussed which never arise, that harm is not balanced by any benefit. Benefit occurs only if the scenario which actually comes to pass has been discussed so that something is known of the patient's preference in that situation. This contrasts with the consent process, whereby patients require only that information which pertains to the current real and necessary decision.

The Joint guidance notes that writing clinically relevant, valid and applicable ACP documents is difficult; various studies showed that only between 10 and 62% of ACP documents relating to hospital treatment contained sufficient information to direct care. Prior discussion with the professional who later has to make the relevant decisions was found to improve the accuracy of interpreting the patient's wishes. But that discussion must entail disclosure of the necessary substantial amount of potentially distressing information—this difficulty is inescapable. Furthermore, if ACP were to be instigated routinely, for example at annual review of patients with long-term conditions as the Joint guidance advises, the treatment options for a wide range of possible (but unpredictable and unknowable) future scenarios would potentially have to be considered.

For the patient, there are risks relating to disclosure of information in the ACP process. The nature and amount of information may be overwhelming, causing distress. But if information is withheld, it is much more likely that an ADRT or an advance statement will not apply in the future circumstances, either because the patient was not well enough informed to envisage the actual scenario which later occurs, or because there were important factors of which the patient was unaware when the ADRT was made, and which would have affected the decision. Insufficient information about likely future circumstances and consequences of decisions can render an ACP discussion at best valueless, and at worst misleading because the preferences recorded are not those the patient would have established if adequately informed.

The ethically difficult judgement for the professional is whether to initiate ACP regarding treatment options, knowing the nature of the information that the patient will require in order to be able to establish preferences. The EoLCP guidance reminds professionals that they should instigate ACP *only if* their judgement leads them to believe it is likely to benefit the patient. To make such a judgement professionals must weigh up the possible benefits of ACP against the harms and risks of contemplating future illness scenarios and ways of dying.

7.5 Professional responsibility for establishing validity and applicability

The broad purpose of advance statements and advance care plans is to know, when capacity has been lost, the choices which the patient would have wanted and which the patient has attempted to communicate in the statement. Patients making ADRTs are attempting to formulate a legally binding refusal of specific treatment(s).

In the case of ADRTs (and arguably also for advance statements/advance care plans), the professional who is the decision-maker when the patient has lost capacity has both a moral and a legal responsibility to establish whether the document (or statement recorded in the notes) is valid, and whether it truly applies to the circumstances which have arisen. The Mental Capacity Act Code of Practice explains the grounds for judging that an apparent ADRT is invalid or inapplicable.[18] These grounds would apply equally to judgements about validity and applicability of advance statements/advance care plans, so the Act is effectively providing professional guidance that is ethically appropriate and necessary. The Joint guidance also notes that an ACP document may be judged invalid.

An advance decision (ADRT) would be invalid if any of the following circumstances pertained. First, if the patient had withdrawn the decision while still having capacity to do so. Second, if, since making the advance decision, the patient had appointed a lasting power of attorney (LPA) giving the attorney authority to make treatment decisions which are the same as those covered by the advance decision. Third, if the patient has done something that clearly goes against the advance decision which suggests a change of mind.

An ADRT would be inapplicable if any of the following circumstances pertained. First, if the proposed treatment is not that specified in the advance decision. Second, if the circumstances are different from those set out in the advance decision. Third, if there are reasonable grounds for believing that there have been changes in circumstance, which would have affected the decision if the person had known about them at the time they made the advance decision.

If an apparent advance decision is judged to be either invalid or inapplicable it is not legally binding, but there is both a moral and a legal duty to consider it as part of the assessment of the patient's best interests, so long as the professionals have reasonable grounds to think that it is a true expression of the person's wishes.

We shall consider first the professional responsibility to establish validity. If the professionals have been caring for the patient in the terminal illness, and particularly if they have been involved in ACP discussions, it will be easier to be satisfied that the patient had not withdrawn the statement/decision, had not appointed an attorney to make the decision, and had capacity when the statement/decision was made. But it can be much more difficult to decide whether the person acted so inconsistently with the advance statement/decision as to render it invalid.

For example, a patient might write an advance statement/care plan or an ADRT indicating that he would not want certain life-prolonging treatments in the context of known terminal illness. But if, having written the statement and while retaining capacity, he chose to undertake those treatments to prolong life (such as antibiotics for infection) then professionals have to judge whether this constitutes an action which is so inconsistent with the previous advance statement/care plan or ADRT as to render it invalid later when he has lost capacity. Furthermore, patients are very unlikely to be aware that acting in a way which is inconsistent with an advance statement/care plan or ADRT, while they retain capacity, may cause professionals to judge that it is invalid when they have lost capacity. The only way to avoid this eventuality is for patients to review their advance statements/care plans and ADRTs regularly, reaffirming them when necessary. This is a complex issue which is difficult to explain to patients.

Judgements about validity are even more difficult when professionals caring for a patient who lacks capacity are faced with an advance statement or ADRT which was written before the present illness and when the patient's circumstances were very different, possibly years earlier. If ACP is encouraged routinely, for example at annual review, or in response to certain recommended triggers, for example bereavement, this scenario will become more frequent.

We shall turn now to the professional responsibility to establish applicability. The most difficult judgement here is whether there have been changes in circumstances (including both clinical and personal circumstances) which would have affected the decision if the person had known about them at the time of making the advance decision. It is, in practice, extremely difficult to know whether the changes in circumstance would have affected the person's decision.

One significant problem for patients is that the more circumstances they specify in an ADRT the less likely it is that it will be legally binding, since it fails to be legally binding if the circumstances specified do not match those which later arise. The Act itself rules that an apparent ADRT will be inapplicable if *any* of the circumstances stipulated in the advance decision are absent.[19] Advance statements/care plans entail similar ethical problems. Patients are faced with conflicting priorities; the more they describe the circumstances in which they would or would not want certain treatment or care measures (so as to make their wishes better understood), the less likely it will be that the circumstances which do later occur will match those specified in the statement or ADRT. But failure to stipulate circumstances makes their wishes less clear to others, and their statement or ADRT may not be interpreted as they would have wished.

We note again that even though the legal stipulations regarding establishment of validity and applicability relate to ADRTs, the ethical issues also extend to advance statements/ACP documents.

There is an argument in favour of laws requiring professionals to assume responsibility for establishing validity and applicability. It is to the effect that professionals can protect patients from the potentially adverse effects of their advance choices. That protection comes into effect if the advance decision (or perhaps advance statement) is judged invalid or inapplicable in the circumstances which arise. But there are three arguments against expecting health care professionals to take this responsibility.

The first relates to fairness in allocation of responsibility. The patient's responsibility is limited to recording the choices (in a particular written format in relation to ADRTs refusing life-prolonging treatment) and for ensuring that the advance statement/care plan or ADRT is accessible when it is needed. By contrast, the professional responsibility to establish validity and applicability is very grave, especially when decisions pertain to life-prolonging treatment, and laws reflect this. For example, the Mental Capacity Act Code of Practice states: 'Before healthcare professionals can apply an advance decision, there must be proof that it exists, is valid, and is applicable in the current circumstances.'[20] It is arguably unfair on professionals to ask them to take the ethically and legally significant responsibility of establishing such 'proof.'

The professional responsibility for establishing validity extends far beyond that which attaches to persons entrusted with carrying out the deceased's wishes expressed in a last will and testament. A will is not invalidated because the maker acted inconsistently with it in life! Nevertheless, professionals are expected to judge whether an advance decision is invalid because a patient acted inconsistently with it while still retaining capacity. It can be argued that patients should be held responsible for ensuring that what they express in ADRTs and advance statements/ACP documents is consistent with their most recent wishes regarding care and treatment in the event of loss of capacity.

With regard to applicability, we have already noted the difficulty of deciding whether an advance decision (or an advance statement/care plan) should be declared inapplicable due to circumstances not foreseen by the patient. Such changes include changes in the patient's 'personal life'.[21] Presumably this could include marriage or divorce, or having had children, or having dependent close relatives. It may be very difficult or impossible to know whether the unforeseen circumstances would have altered the advance decision had the patient been aware of them. This is even more problematic if the advance decision/statement was written before the present illness or years earlier.

The ethically important point is that the responsibility for the very difficult decisions on validity and applicability is onerous for health care professionals, who may even be exposed to litigation or threat of litigation if others (such as family members) feel that they made an error of judgement.

The second argument against giving to health care professionals the responsibility for establishing 'proof' of validity and applicability is, ironically, that it then becomes rather too easy for them to find reasons why an advance decision or statement should be declared invalid or inapplicable. Indeed, it is sometimes noted that in the context of an actual clinical situation it is almost always possible to find some grounds to declare an apparent ADRT invalid or inapplicable! Since 'proof' is difficult to establish there may be a natural tendency to declare the advance decision invalid or inapplicable. Once so declared, it is no longer legally binding. It has to be taken into account, but will be completely overridden if the professional judges that following the advance decision would not be in the best interests of the patient. The same problems apply to some extent to advance statements/care plans, in that it is relatively easy to find reasons why they may not be valid or applicable.

The third argument against allocating this responsibility to professionals is that costs will be charged to the National Health Service (NHS) if it has to apply for legal advice or a court decision. There is an argument for passing to the patient's legal representatives the responsibility for establishing validity and applicability, and for passing the costs to the patient rather than to the NHS.

Such an arrangement would more closely reflect the socially sanctioned system for administration of wills.

To sum up the ethical issues, we can say that whereas patients are being encouraged to make advance choices, they are not expected to take full responsibility for those choices (yet we normally associate choice with responsibility for that choice). Instead, much responsibility passes to health care professionals. Readers are left to judge whether the three arguments against this policy are persuasive. If so, they may conclude that the fact that the patient is making 'advance' choices should not remove from the patient so much responsibility for those choices.

7.6 **Importance of recording and review**

Review is important because it ensures that what is stated reflects the patient's most recent preferences, and a recent review date reassures professionals and patients' families that this is the case. The Joint guidance group found evidence that up to one-third of patients will change their advance statement over a time period of months to years, influenced by changes not only in diagnosis and health status but also in mood, hospitalization, functional ability and social circumstances.

There is also an argument for suggesting review if the patient has acted inconsistently with respect to the statement while capacity is retained, since such action might indicate a change of mind, in which case the statement should be revised. As we explained in the previous section, dated review after an action inconsistent with the statement helps to prevent professionals from judging that the statement should be regarded as invalid.

The two ACP documents recommended nationally in the UK (*Preferred priorities for care* and Gold Standards Framework (GSF) Centre's *Thinking ahead*) prompt patients to review their preferences.[22,23] The EoLCP guidance recommends that the record of the ACP discussion should state clearly when a review is planned, and that review might be instigated by the professional, perhaps as part of a regular review policy or triggered by a change in the patient's circumstances.

The ethical problem for professionals is whether or how often to instigate review. One might suggest that they should do this whenever there is a significant change in the patient's clinical condition. But in end of life care it could be burdensome for patients to be asked to review their preferences every time their condition worsened, since a review necessarily entails contemplating again the future illness scenarios. It might even appear that the professionals were suggesting that, following a clinical deterioration, the patient might no longer want life-prolonging treatment in the event of loss of capacity, or might want a different location of care.

Readers are left to judge what policies they think should be followed with regard to instigation of review by professionals, including whether this should be according to a pre-planned time schedule, a change in the patient's condition such as reduced functional ability or hospitalization, or perhaps even a change noted in the patient's mood and social circumstances.

7.7 Responsibility for taking advance statements into account in best interests judgements

Ethically relevant guidance on this issue is given in the Mental Capacity Act Code of Practice.[24] It states that 'The decision-maker should consider written statements carefully. If their decision does not follow something a person has put in writing, they must record the reasons why. They should be able to justify their reasons if someone challenges their decision.' With regard to requests for treatment, it states 'A doctor should take written statements which request specific treatment as seriously as those made by people who currently have capacity to make treatment decisions. But they would not have to follow a written request if they think the specific treatment would be clinically unnecessary or not appropriate for the person's condition, so not in the person's best interests.'

Although this guidance sounds ethically entirely reasonable, professionals concerned about the possibility of complaints and litigation might judge that they will be less open to criticism if they comply with patients' advance choices. But there will undoubtedly be times when complying with those choices will actually be contrary to patients' best interests. Whereas patients have been enabled to express advance choices, all the responsibility for acting on those choices passes to the professionals (unless the patient has made a legally binding ADRT).

Advance statements, including ACP documents, may contain statements about values, goals or desired outcomes rather than preferences regarding identified treatments. The Joint guidance group found that patients preferred this option, but professionals found such statements more difficult to interpret. For example, patients describing themselves as a 'fighter' will leave others unclear about what they would want to 'fight' for. So statements about goals, values and beliefs may not influence decisions in the way which patients might wish. Is there duty to advise patients of this difficulty?

7.8 Ethically important common misunderstandings

As with many new policies and interventions, misunderstandings and errors are likely. ACP is no exception. We shall discuss five common, and ethically important, misunderstandings.

7.8.i **Failure to distinguish ACP from other forms of care planning**

It is common for ACP to be confused with care planning more generally. For example, whilst the *End of life care strategy* refers to ACP and the relevant national guidance it does not make clear that its purpose is to guide decision-making if the patient loses capacity in the future.[25] Furthermore, it does not make it clear that so long as the patient retains capacity it must be the patient's contemporaneous views which are elicited and which carry weight, not the contents of an advance statement; a clinical example given unfortunately reinforces the confusion. The Strategy otherwise generally refers to 'care plans' rather than advance care plans/statements.

Neither of the two ACP documents recommended nationally in the UK make it clear to patients that the purpose of ACP is to aid decision-making if they should lose capacity, and that advance statements such as these documents should not be used in decision-making so long as capacity is retained.

Advance care planning is also sometimes referred to as 'Advanced' care planning. This is not a typographical error, it expresses a profound misunderstanding. Its ethical importance lies in the fact that it implies that ACP is a form of 'super care planning', and the error actually obfuscates the true nature of the intervention.

Current misunderstanding is ethically important because patients may not adequately comprehend why they are being asked to complete an ACP document, or to sanction a record of the discussion made by a professional. If they do not comprehend the purpose of ACP they may not ascribe sufficient importance to expressing and recording preferences. They might even think that professionals could disregard their recorded preferences if those preferences did not accord with their best interests at the time. But this belief is false—the law understandably insists that decision-makers must take account of recorded preferences.

7.8.ii **Failure to recognize the importance of voluntariness**

The EoLCP guidance on ACP, the evidence-based Joint guidance on ACP and the *End of life care strategy* all make it clear that the process of ACP is voluntary for the patient. The first states that 'No pressure should be brought to bear by the professional, the family or any organization on the individual concerned to take part in ACP.' Arguably, pressure to engage in ACP is a form of abuse. A non-UK survey of cancer patients, healthy controls, and medical staff showed that more than one-third of those who felt their health was tolerable or poor, and more than one-half of those who felt well, feared abuse of 'advance directives' by relatives.[26]

Despite professional guidance, subtle pressure is sometimes brought to bear on patients for three reasons. The first is a genuine belief in the value of ACP for the patient. The second is organizational or professional pressure to achieve the patient's previously expressed choice in terms of place of death; if the extent of that achievement is to be audited, perhaps as some sort of performance measurement/target, then patients must take part in ACP. The third is a desire of professionals to make easier their own task of forming best interests judgements for the patients once capacity is lost; knowing the patient's previously expressed views can make the process easier, and the decision made easier to defend if it is questioned.

Whilst these reasons explain why patients might be put under pressure, however subtle, they do not justify such pressure.

7.8.iii Failure to recognize the patient's right to confidentiality

The 2008 PPC document explains that it might be helpful to discuss the PPC with your family and friends and indeed encourages this, but does not explicitly state that it is quite possible and acceptable to keep the discussion and PPC document confidential and not divulge its contents to family and friends.

The GSF ACP discussion record, *Thinking ahead*, informs patients that the aim of ACP 'is to develop a better understanding and recording of their priorities, needs and preferences and those of their families/carers.' This statement clearly implies that the aim of the exercise is to ascertain the preferences of families and other carers, not just those of the patient. So confidentiality for the patient seems to be at best irrelevant and at worst virtually excluded as a possibility!

Such inadequate regard for patients' right to confidentiality may be due to the belief that involving the family in the ACP discussion helps to ensure that patient and family share the same insight into the patient's clinical situation. Involving the family in the discussion may also foster discussion and hopefully agreement between patient and family regarding the care that the latter are willing and able to provide at home. The difficulty of arranging an interview with the patient alone may also compromise confidentiality.

Once again, although these reasons provide explanations, they cannot justify the practice of failing to ensure that the patient is aware of the possibility of a confidential discussion and record, and that families of patients are not included in the ACP discussion unless the patient so wishes.

Confidentiality is also an issue regarding disclosure to all professionals making decisions—advance statements cannot be effective unless decision-makers have access to them when decisions are needed. But the contents of the statement cannot be disclosed to anyone unless the author of the statement/ care plan has agreed to disclosure, as the EoLCP guidance rightly stipulates. That guidance advises that where patients decline disclosure the options should be explained to them and the consequences made clear. Patients face an inescapable conflict between confidentiality and accessibility of the statement. The *End of life care strategy* fails to acknowledge this problem when instructing that 'care plans, including the person's preferences, wishes and views on resuscitation, should be available to all who have a legitimate reason to access them, including out of hours and emergency/urgent care services. Holding the plan electronically will facilitate this.'[27] It is the right and responsibility of patients to make the statement/care plan available to those professionals whom they choose, but this may not be understood either by patients or professionals, leading to breaches of confidentiality or lack of availability of the statements/ ACP documents when they are needed.

7.8.iv Failure to obtain the patient's permission to record the outcome of the ACP discussion

This problem arises if the outcome of the discussion is recorded by the professional in the health care records. Professionals may simply not appreciate the requirement to ask the patient's permission before making a record of the outcome of the discussion. Clinicians are not accustomed to explicitly agreeing with patients what is written in health care records, and it may prove difficult to persuade them that they have this ethical obligation in this instance. Patients might also find the process rather legalistic. But if professionals and patients did understand this issue there would be better appreciation of the importance and potentially serious consequences of the entire exercise of ACP.

7.8.v Misunderstandings regarding the function of advance statements, advance care plans in best interests judgements

As we note in Chapter 8, much importance is now attached to patients dying in the place of their choice, and, as many patients lose capacity prior to death, the 'choice' is frequently that which has been expressed in advance. The two ACP documents recommended in the UK both specifically ask about preference for location of care. This issue is similarly stressed in the *End of life care strategy*.[28] The emphasis on achievement of the patient's advance choice of place of care, and particularly death, might lead professionals to believe that this choice is the most important factor in a best interests judgement.

Similarly, patients, their families and professionals might be led to believe that treatment preferences recorded in an advance statement are the overriding factor in best interests judgements.

But this is not the case either ethically or legally. For example, the Mental Capacity Act stipulates that 'all the relevant circumstances' should be considered in such a best interests judgement, not just what can be known of the patient's wishes.[29] This stipulation appears ethically not just reasonable but necessary, since professionals must consider the balance of benefit to harm and risk for the various treatment/care options, and not merely the preference stated in advance.

For example, a patient might have recorded in an advance statement/advance care plan that she did not want readmission to hospital. But if she then develops confusion secondary to infection or adverse reaction to medication, which could be most effectively treated during a brief hospital stay, it may well be in her best interests to be admitted for a short period. Rigorous adherence to her advance statement may not coincide with her best interests.

Disproportionate stress placed on achieving patients' advance choices may lead professionals to act contrary to the best interests of patients lacking capacity. It may also cause patients to develop unrealistic expectations. Both outcomes are ethically highly undesirable.

Putting aside the potential for these misunderstandings, we can now consider the basic moral argument in favour of advance statements/advance care plans.

7.9 Support for ACP, advance statements

In the latter part of the twentieth century both health care ethics and the philosophy of palliative care emphasized the importance of respecting and enhancing the patient's 'autonomy'. Autonomy here was used in the sense of the patient's self-determination or ability to make choices. Advance statements, and more recently ACP, have been regarded as ways to extend choice into that time when capacity is lost. The question then arises as to whether patients ought to be encouraged, or routinely requested, to undertake ACP followed by a recorded statement, including an ADRT if desired. Professional guidance already recommends that in certain circumstances patients should be asked whether they would/would not wish CPR to be attempted. In end of life care, should ACP be instigated as a matter of routine in relation to other potentially life-prolonging treatments, when it is foreseen that a decision may be needed at a time when the patient may lack capacity?

We have noted in Section 7.1 that ACP is a health care intervention which is being driven forwards at national level via NHS policy, guidance, and possibly by future performance measures. There is currently also a strong political agenda directed towards promoting patient choice, which would clearly extend to making choices in advance of the occassion when they will be applied. If we are to ask patients to undertake ACP and make advance statements we must be clear about our motivation in so doing. This requires consideration of the arguments in favour of, and arguments against, this intervention; in the foregoing discussion we have drawn attention to the advantages of ACP, to some potential disadvantages, and also to the ethical problems inherent in its implementation.

7.10 **ACP: an intervention with a limited UK evidence base**

Advance care planning should be recognized as a health care intervention when instigated by a health care professional. The justifications for so doing are that it is voluntary for the patient but requires professional activity, and whereas it may bestow benefits it also has the potential to cause harms, and risks are entailed in interpreting and implementing advance statements. It is also relevant that it is not necessary for current decision-making with the patient who has capacity (but it can be undertaken only when the patient retains capacity). Furthermore, it is currently promoted as an intervention, and guidance for professionals has been produced to try to ensure that it is correctly carried out in clinical practice. Failure to follow this guidance, and thus improper clinical practice, would be a clinical governance issue.

It is also a health care intervention with potentially very widespread application—all patients will ultimately die, and the great majority of adults will have capacity and therefore the ability to carry out ACP, even if this might be years before their final illness and death. In terms of its scope of application to very large numbers of the population it compares with the largest major national screening programmes.

But the intervention of ACP has been promoted nationally without much experience of it in the UK, and without much UK evidence. This was noted by the group who searched the evidence base in producing the Joint guidance. Their grading of the evidence demonstrates that little of it is of the highest quality and much of it is graded only as expert opinion from users or professionals. Furthermore, they commented that most of the evidence that does exist is from North America and they noted that it should be interpreted with much caution in the UK context. Fewer than 10 of the 140 publications they found were from work done in the UK (personal communication).

So we do not currently have the evidence to know the overall balance of benefit to harm and risk for patients as a result of this intervention in the UK, even when it is carried out according to recent national guidance. What we do know is that, even if properly carried out, ACP is associated with practical difficulties which are inevitable and are ethically significant.

We have drawn attention to common (and dangerous) misunderstandings about its nature, purpose and implementation in clinical practice. These are ethically very significant. With regard to ACP documents, the Joint guidance group found that none of the 12 they reviewed was ideal, and we have noted individual problems with the UK-promoted PPC and GSF documents. The shortcomings of ACP documents perpetuate misunderstandings about the intervention, increasing the likelihood of harm and risk to patients from attempts at implementation.

At present we do not have the evidence to inform us whether the widespread introduction of ACP into our health care system, and the routine offer of ACP to patients in the contexts of long-term conditions and end of life care, will provide overall benefit to patients or overall harm and risk. There may of course be a difference in the outcomes of ACP when it is used in the context of end of life care, as opposed to when it is used by patients not currently suffering from a life-limiting disease.

We also do not know the resource consequences. Resources will be required for the education and training of health care professionals, for the ACP discussions between patients and professionals, and for the provision of treatment and care which patients state in advance that they would want, including the preferred place of care and death.

It is perhaps puzzling that the intervention of ACP has been promoted nationally on the basis of so little evidence about its net benefit or otherwise to large numbers of patients, and about its costs in terms of money and manpower. It is worth comparing the introduction of ACP with that of screening programmes—the latter are not introduced without careful scrutiny of the balance of benefit to harm and risk, and detailed analysis of the costs and cost-effectiveness. Doubt has been cast on the wisdom of introducing health care interventions without an adequate evidence base.[30] In a publicly funded health care system, and given the intrinsic vulnerability of patients to interventions advocated in that system (especially in end of life care), it is a matter of ethical importance that ACP has been promoted without the knowledge base which has rightly been deemed essential before widespread promotion of other comparable interventions.

To highlight some of the ethical problems of ACP we shall consider a specific clinical treatment decision (CPR), because it is the only treatment for which

ACP is deemed essential in specific circumstances. In Chapter 8 we shall examine another controversial aspect of ACP—the 'preferred place of care and death' policy.

7.11 Cardiopulmonary resuscitation and ACP

The most recent UK professional guidance on decision-making relating to CPR, issued jointly by the BMA, Resuscitation Council and Royal College of Nursing in October 2007, states in its main messages that 'Advance care planning, including making decisions about cardiopulmonary resuscitation, is an important part of good clinical care for those at risk of cardiorespiratory arrest.'[31]

Clearly, in the context of end of life care the majority of patients are at risk of cardiorespiratory arrest, and indeed this event is inevitable at death. The guidance on CPR helpfully explains that where it has no realistic prospect of success, in terms of restarting the heart and breathing for a sustained period, it should not be attempted. This instruction is clear and uncontroversial. But the guidance is controversial in respect of patients in whom CPR might succeed.

There will be some circumstances in end of life in which CPR will have a realistic prospect of success. For example, a patient with incurable cancer may still be up and about, leading a fairly normal life, but may then suffer cardiorespiratory arrest due to an arrhythmia secondary to a myocardial infarction. CPR might then be successful, especially in a coronary care unit. But the harms and risks of attempting CPR are significant, rates of survival to leave hospital are generally low, and in end of life care patients are further disadvantaged by comorbidities.

The guidance suggests that where cardiorespiratory arrest is foreseen and CPR might be effective, and 'where the expected benefit may be outweighed by the burdens, the patient's informed views are of paramount importance.' It therefore effectively recommends that in the context of end of life care, for those patients in whom CPR would have a realistic prospect of success, health care staff definitely should instigate ACP regarding CPR. The aim is then to determine and record whether or not the patient would want CPR to be attempted in the event of cardiopulmonary arrest, and perhaps the clinical circumstances in which the patient would wish the stated preferences to apply.

For example, some patients would want CPR to be attempted if they had been independent and comfortable immediately prior to cardiorespiratory arrest, but not if they had irreversibly lost capacity to make most decisions in life, were largely unable to communicate and were dependent on others for care. These scenarios might be envisaged by a patient with very early Alzheimer's disease.

Although the guidance instructs professionals to instigate ACP discussions about CPR in these circumstances, patients can decline to take part and such a refusal must be respected. But what is ethically interesting about the case of CPR is that this is the only medical treatment decision which we are told patients should specifically be asked to consider in advance, and then to leave a record of their wishes. Is this policy justified?

There are plausible reasons to support such a policy, although some contest whether they adequately justify asking patients to engage in ACP regarding CPR attempts in the context of end of life care.[32] The argument rests upon the following particular features of CPR as a treatment: there is no time for a considered best interests judgement at cardiorespiratory arrest, so any properly considered decision must be made in advance; CPR is unusual in that there is a presumption in favour of attempting it if no prior DNAR (do not attempt resuscitation) decision has been made; CPR has a low success rate, especially in terms of achieving discharge from hospital afterwards; CPR has significant associated harms and risks—it is an invasive and undignified procedure, many patients never return to their previous fitness after a successful attempt, and there is a small but real risk of survival with hypoxic brain damage which can be severe.

The operation of all these factors together results in a situation whereby, unless a DNAR decision has been made in advance, the patient in whom CPR might be successful will be subjected to it. But it is clear that there are many situations where the expected benefit may be outweighed by the burdens, hence the guidance that the patient's informed views are paramount in deciding whether attempting CPR is in the patient's best interests. The only way to avoid unwanted CPR attempts is to seek patients' views in ACP discussions, and (with the patient's permission) to record the outcome of such discussion.

Readers may judge for themselves whether or not they feel that this chain of argument justifies the current guidance and policies derived from it. Some might conclude that, in the context of end of life care, it would have been preferable to abandon the presumption in favour of CPR where no decision has been made in advance.

7.12 Conclusions

1) Advance care planning is a complex and relatively new health care intervention for which further evaluation, especially in the UK context, is required.

2) If national guidance is not well understood and adhered to, patients and professionals may misunderstand the process, giving rise to several kinds

of failure: to understand its purpose; to ensure that the process is voluntary for patients; to understand that it is confidential if the patient wishes it so; and to understand its specific role in best interests judgements for patients who lack capacity.

3) Properly conducted, ACP is likely to enable patients' previously stated preferences to be understood and taken into account once they have lost capacity. It may also improve decision-making via the best interests process, and make the tasks of professionals and family members in this process less burdensome.

4) But there are problems inherent in the requirements to assess validity and applicability of both advance decisions to refuse treatment and advance statements/care plans. Interpretation of advance statements can be difficult, leading to interpretations that the patient may not have intended.

5) There is a risk that the ACP process may give rise to unrealistic patient expectations and in some patients to avoidable emotional distress.

References

1. British Medical Association (1993). *Medical ethics today.* BMJ Books, London, pp. 161–4.
2. UK Government (2005). Mental Capacity Act 2005. Office of Public Sector Information, London.
3. Department for Constitutional Affairs (2007). Mental Capacity Act 2005 Code of Practice. The Stationery Office, Norwich, pp. 158–76.
4. National Institute for Clinical Excellence (2004). *Improving supportive and palliative care for adults with cancer.* NICE, London, pp. 118–19.
5. Department of Health (2008). *End of life care strategy.* DoH, London, pp. 53–4.
6. General Medical Council (2008). *Consent: patients and doctors making decisions together.* GMC, London, para. 57–61.
7. *R (Burke)* v *General Medical Council* (defendant) and *Disability Rights Commission* (interested party) and the *Official Solicitor* (intervenor) [2004] EWHC 1879.
8. Mohindra R (2006). Obligations to treat, personal autonomy, and artificial nutrition and hydration. *Clinical Medicine* **6**:271–3.
9. Samanta A, Samanta J (2006). Advance directives, best interests and clinical judgement: shifting sands at the end of life. *Clinical Medicine* **6**:274–8.
10. DCA, op. cit. (ref. 3), pp. 81–2.
11. End of Life Care Programme (2008). *Advance care planning: a guide for health and social care staff.* Available at http://www.endoflifecare.nhs.uk (accessed on 16.1.09).
12. End of Life Care Programme, op. cit. (ref. 11).
13. Royal College of Physicians, National Council for Palliative Care, British Society of Rehabilitation Medicine, British Geriatrics Society, Alzheimer's Society, Royal College of Nursing, Royal College of Psychiatrists, Help the Aged, Royal College of General

Practitioners (2009). *Advance care planning*. Concise Guidance to Good Practice series, No. 12. Royal College of Physicians, London.

14. Conroy S, Fade P, Fraser A, Schiff R (2009). Advance care planning: concise evidence-based guidelines. *Clinical Medicine* **9**:76–9.

15. Department of Health (2008). *Advance decisions to refuse treatment: a guide for health and social care professionals*. Available at http://www.adrtnhs.co.uk (accessed 16.1.09).

16. GMC, op. cit. (ref. 6), para. 57.

17. Department of Health, op. cit. (ref. 5), p. 6.

18. DCA, op. cit. (ref. 3), pp. 169–74.

19. UK Government, op. cit. (ref. 2), section 25 (4).

20. DCA, op. cit. (ref. 3), p. 160.

21. DCA, op. cit. (ref. 3), p. 171.

22. National PPC Review Team (2007). *Preferred priorities for care*. Available at http://www.endoflifecareforadults.nhs.uk/eolc/ppc.htm (accessed on 16.1.09).

23. Gold Standards Framework Centre (2008). *Thinking ahead—advance care planning discussion*. Available at http://www.goldstandardsframework.nhs.uk/advanced_care.php (accessed 16.1.09).

24. DCA, op. cit. (ref. 3), pp. 80–82.

25. Department of Health, op. cit. (ref. 5), p. 54.

26. Sahm S, Will R, Hommel G (2005). Attitudes towards and barriers to writing advance directives amongst cancer patients, healthy controls, and medical staff. *Journal of Medical Ethics* **31**:437–440.

27. Department of Health, op. cit. (ref. 5), p. 57.

28. Department of Health, op. cit. (ref. 5), p. 17.

29. DCA, op. cit. (ref. 3), pp. 74–5.

30. Landefeld CS, Shojania KG, Auerbach AD (2008). Should we use large scale healthcare interventions without clear evidence that benefits outweigh costs and harms? *BMJ* **336**:1276–7.

31. British Medical Association, Resuscitation Council (UK), Royal College of Nursing (2007). *Decisions relating to cardiopulmonary resuscitation*. BMA, London.

32. Regnard C, Randall F (2009). Should hospices be exempt from following national cardiopulmonary resuscitation guidelines? No. *BMJ* **338**:b986.

Preferred place of care and death

In recent years increasing stress has been placed on the importance of ensuring that patients' preferences for location of care, particularly death, are achieved. Advance care planning documents include preferred place of care as a specific question. But has too much emphasis now been placed on this one aspect of care? We felt that this issue merits consideration. We refer to the policy of attributing very high or overriding priority to patients dying in the place of their choice as the 'preferred place of care and death' policy.

8.1 The national context

Many people will retain capacity until very close to death, and loss of capacity will not be expected in their case. So discussions with them are part of care planning generally, rather than advance care planning (ACP) for anticipated loss of capacity. Whether place of care and death is a matter of normal care planning, or a topic in ACP, meeting patients' preferences in this regard does raise some major ethical issues.

Much of the emphasis on achieving the patient's choice for place of death originated in the context of specialist palliative care. In 2004 the World Health Organization expressed the view that meeting people's preferences for place of care and death should be 'the ultimate measure of success' for a service.[1] Also in that year the National Institute for Clinical Excellence (NICE) guidance recommended the ACP Preferred Place of Care document (now withdrawn).[2] This ACP document had an audit function to ascertain the extent to which patients' preferences for place of death had been achieved. The NICE guidance also recommended adoption of the Gold Standards Framework (GSF)—its ACP document specifically asks about the patient's preferences regarding place of care.

The *End of life care strategy* reports that large scale surveys to assess public attitudes to death and dying have shown that 'most people would prefer to die at home'.[3] We would add here the caveat that the great majority of people questioned in such surveys would not actually be receiving end of life care and thus facing the options in reality. Clearly one cannot assume that preferences expressed by the public in general would necessarily be the same as those of patients facing the choices in reality. The strategy emphasizes throughout the aim of achieving patients' choices, but it is balanced in that it also emphasizes the aims of achieving high quality care wherever the patient is, of equality, and of value for money.[4]

The two sets of UK guidance on ACP for health care professionals (End of Life Care Programme and evidence-based Joint guidance, see Section 7.1) do not advocate specifically questioning patients about their preferred place of care and/or death.

But the political picture is rather different. A great deal of stress has been placed on achieving the patient's choice for place of death. Alan Johnson, the then Secretary of State for Health, is reported to have said of the *End of life care strategy*: 'The priority is to improve community services to enable all adults, regardless of their condition, to die in the setting of their choice.'[5] We should here note that the Strategy's aims, as mentioned above, are much broader and more balanced than this statement implies.

In England, the South West Strategic Health Authority has gone even further, ambitiously stating that 'We will develop end of life care plans with patients to ensure that they are able to die peacefully and with dignity, free from pain and fear, in a setting of their choice, with relatives and loved ones'. It included in its improvements in care that 'All health communities to be able by 31 March 2011 to be able to identify the number of people with a plan for their death and to report the percentage of cases where the preference about place of death has been achieved.' It therefore naturally also recommended that organizations involved in end of life care should use 'care plans as an audit tool'.[6] Other health authorities are likely to follow in making audit a primary purpose of care planning, as we explain in Section 8.2.iv.

Specialist palliative care has traditionally stressed the importance of eliciting the patient's preferences for place of care and death and achieving these where possible. But recently Dr Julia Riley, a consultant in palliative medicine, went much further in an editorial in the *BMJ*.[7] She recommended that specialists in palliative medicine should monitor continuously the percentage of patients who died in the place of their choice. She recommended that they should focus on this percentage, 'perhaps on "personal dashboards", which show in real time what is happening in terms of performance'. The analogy of keeping one's eyes on a dial on a car dashboard as one is driving is certainly interest-ing—it raises the question of how safe one's performance would be, either in driving the car or in clinical care! Her hope was that specialists might be further urged to increase this percentage, spurred on by a competitive spirit to achieve a better 'performance' than their colleagues! She went on to recom-mend that the patient's wishes and care plan should be available at every contact with the service, and stated without qualification that 'Whenever an intervention of any sort occurs in primary care, secondary care, community services, or social services the patient's exact wishes must be known and complied with.'

In a later letter to the *BMJ* Dr Riley recommended that patients' preferences should be recorded contemporaneously on an 'electronic, summary care record for palliative care patients that will be accessible to all specialist and generic professionals including the out of hours service'.[8] The English health authority mentioned above similarly recommended availability of plans at all times. Such statements completely fail to acknowledge the importance of enabling patients to keep personal preferences/plans confidential if they wish, and their right to do so. All seems to have been sacrificed on the altar of achieving the patient's choice in terms of place of death! The ethical problems and functional limits of clinical dashboards were highlighted in a subsequent letter to the *BMJ*, where it was noted that when targets on dashboards are not met 'excuses are followed by the realisation that some of the targets are unachievable, even undesirable.'[9]

It is essential to ask what might be sacrificed if patients' preferences for place of death are to be sought, known, and complied with. One can then consider whether the value of achieving patients' preferences, almost come-what-may, outweighs the other values which are very likely to be compromised as a result. Those other values are considered now, and for ease of discussion are numbered below.

8.2 Ethical problems arising from preferred place of care and death policy

8.2.i Voluntariness in ACP and care planning generally

If patients' preferences are to be achieved, they must be known. So a vigorous and concerted attempt to achieve their preferences is likely to result in pressure on all patients identified as approaching the end of their lives to answer a specific question about where they want to die. A more tactful question about their preference for place of care (as in the current Preferred Priorities for Care and GSF ACP documents) would not suffice because a significant proportion of patients want most of their care to be at home, but they do not want to die there.[10] For example, evidence-based data quoted by the National Council for Palliative Care in 2002 indicated that about 25% of patients actually want to die in 'a hospice'.[11]

Political pressures, plus a desire for 'outcome measures', are likely to lead to targets and 'performance measures' or 'metrics' regarding this one goal. This is an almost inevitable development since the event and location of death are known (whereas other outcome measures are difficult to devise for end of life care as so little of it is 'measurable'). Of course the remaining factor for this outcome measure is the patient's preference. So using the percentage of patients achieving their preferred place of death as a 'performance/outcome' measure is extremely likely to lead to pressure on patients to engage in discussions and record their preference (in advance) for place of death. For example, the health authority cited above fails to acknowledge that such planning for death should be voluntary for patients.

The imperative that such discussions must be voluntary is essential to protect patients from being urged into planning the location of their death at a time when they are unready or unwilling to confront the issues. Patients vary in their ability and desire to plan for their own death—some will never wish to engage in ACP for death. If they are pressurized into such conversations, especially when they are in a vulnerable position relative to the power of the professional on whom they are dependent for care, they are likely to suffer unnecessary emotional harm. The potential for harm resulting from audits where there is such power imbalance was highlighted in a *BMJ* paper on ethics in relation to audit and research.[12] It is to avoid such harm that the national guidance on ACP stipulates so clearly that patients should not be put under any pressure, even for organizational reasons, to undertake ACP (see Sections 7.3 and 7.8.ii).

Sadly, the ethically necessary value of voluntariness in ACP will almost inevitably be sacrificed if achievement of patients' preferred place of death becomes a measure/marker of organizational and professional performance.

8.2.ii Pressure on patients to express achievable preferences

Of course one way in which the goal can most easily be achieved is to ensure that preferences expressed by patients are those which are likely to be achieved. Some preferences are unlikely to be achievable now, or in the foreseeable future.

For example, as stated above it is believed that about 25% of patients would like to die in a hospice. But evidence reveals that only about 4–5% currently do so.[13] There are no plans to significantly increase the availability of hospice/specialist palliative care beds. So if a patient expresses a desire to die in a hospice the staff will know that this is unlikely to be achieved, especially if the patient does not have cancer.[14]

This raises the ethically important question of whether staff should seek the patient's genuine preference and endeavour to ensure that this is recorded, or should seek to influence the patient's stated preference so that it becomes more achievable. The strongest ethical argument for the former is that it allows patients to express freely what is genuinely their preference for their own death. Efforts could then be made to achieve it, even though they might not be successful. The ethical argument in favour of exerting influence is that patients can be brought to understand what is likely to be achievable and what is not, given clinical circumstances and resources, and so patients can be saved from having unrealistic expectations. They can also express a preference based on knowledge of what care facilities are available in different locations and, if relevant, how they are funded.

But if achievement of the patient's recorded preference becomes an extremely important outcome or performance measure, or is seen as clinically of very great importance, then a practical (as opposed to an ethical) imperative will exist to persuade patients to state an achievable preference. Organizational pressure, exerted via health care professionals, would be used to persuade patients to do this.

For example, the health authority strategic framework cited above states that 'NHS South West will expect the practice of having good discussions, resulting in realistic and practical plans agreed with the individual, to be adopted by all organisations.' So this NHS strategic health authority seeks to place on professionals the responsibility for ensuring that the patient agrees to record a preference which is 'realistic and practical', and so likely to be achieved. It is clear that this practice would improve the audit figures regarding patients dying in the place of their recorded preference. It is much less clear that it would really result in patients dying in 'the place of their choice'. It is also debatable whether placing this responsibility on professionals is ethically justifiable.

Ensuring that only preferences likely to be achieved are recorded could reasonably be regarded as 'gaming'. The strategy of gaming to improve results in performance measures is well recognized, and it was noted in an editorial on health policy that 'Systems need to be put in place to minimise gaming to meet targets and ensure that targets are not causing unwanted effects elsewhere.'[15] Limiting patients' ability to express genuine preferences is an ethically unwanted effect!

There are obvious implications here for the wider debate on patient choice in the NHS. We have already noted the differences between the everyday notion of choosing between available options in a pre-determined range, and the notion of consumer choice which is a matter of choosing between all possible options. The question here is whether patients should be presented only with those location options which are achievable (a range determined by the clinical and service circumstances) or whether patients should be permitted to express a preference for any location, be it home, specialist palliative care unit, nursing home or hospital. An expansive interpretation of consumer choice would also include other parts of the UK or even the Bahamas!

8.2.iii Effects on decision-making for patients who lack capacity

Many patients do lose capacity in the period just before death, especially in the last few days when consciousness is often diminishing or lost. We note in Section 7.8.v that professional ethics (and law) require that decisions made for patients who lack capacity must be based only on the patient's best interests; the best interests judgement process requires that all the relevant circumstances be considered, not just whatever can be known of the patient's wishes and feelings, beliefs and values. The relevant circumstances for patients who are imminently dying obviously include their physical and mental condition and the care and treatment options which have the greatest likelihood of alleviating distress, whether physical or mental. What can be known of the patient's wishes, feelings, beliefs and values will have been recorded as the patient's stated preference, or information about them can be gleaned (as far as possible and appropriate) from friends and family.

This decision-making process was established after years of discussion, followed by consultation, and the final consensus is expressed in law relating to patients who lack capacity. We describe it in Section 2.5.

But if great stress is placed on achieving the patient's recorded preference for place of care/death, then this factor will be given much greater sway in the decision. It may even, in practice, come to override all other factors so that a true 'best interests' judgement is no longer made. This is especially likely to occur if professionals are influenced, subtly or overtly, to try to improve the 'outcome/performance measure' figures. Practical results would include some patients remaining in a location which was their previously stated preference but which is not now in their overall best interests, perhaps because adequate care and symptom control are unlikely to be achieved there. Other patients might be moved, when close to death, to that place which was their previously recorded preference.

Readers might object that moribund patients will not be moved around in ambulances in order to meet a performance target. But readers should then reflect on the occasions they will be aware of when clinically inappropriate action has been taken merely to achieve targets, especially when the penalties for falling short of the target were measures ultimately punitive for patients. A thoughtful letter from a junior doctor notes that her 'Trust policy actively ignores clinical guidelines to achieve performance indicators.'[16]

The harms of target-driven care are now being recognized, and were well summarized by Nigel Rawlinson.[17] He noted that 'However hard we try to remain patient focused, meeting targets is now the predominant driver'. His words also echo warnings about the use of targets in the context of end of life care: 'There is now less time for the vulnerable, frightened, and inarticulate patients, who become objects of annoyance rather than subjects of care.' and 'Targets encourage patients to be categorised into management pathways.' It is all too easy to imagine vulnerable and anxious or inarticulate patients being pressurized, however subtly, into making advance statements about their preferred place of death, being discouraged from expressing a preference which is unlikely to be achieved, and then being funnelled down the appropriate 'pathway' to achieve the recorded preference, with insufficient chance to review the options and change their minds.

We should note that in this situation the law could be used by professionals to defend patients against the adverse effects of political and organizational pressures. For example, the Code of Practice for the Mental Capacity Act stipulates that patients' 'wishes and feelings, beliefs and values will not necessarily be the deciding factor in working out their best interests . . . the final decision must be based entirely on what is in the person's best interests.'[18]

Anyone declaring, as Dr Riley did in her editorial in the *BMJ* regarding advance care plans (quoted in Section 8.1), that 'the patient's exact wishes must be known and complied with' is making a statement which is factually incorrect in terms of professional ethics (and UK law) in respect of patients who lack capacity.

8.2.iv **Audit**

If achievement of the patient's preferred place of death is considered to be of great importance, or is to function as an outcome/performance measure, then audits will be necessary to provide data. Audits will first entail collection of patients' advance care plans/care plans at some central point, possibly a primary or secondary care trust. These care plans will have to contain patient identifiers so that each one can be compared with the known place of death, perhaps from death certificates. It is therefore extremely difficult to conduct such large audits anonymously.

We noted in Section 8.1 the aim of one health authority that NHS organizations should know how many people in their area have made an advance care plan regarding place of death, and should also know the percentage in which this was achieved. Both of these requirements would necessitate primary and secondary care trusts collecting and retaining very personal information. The question also arises as to how such organizations could even know if a person not receiving end of life care had made an advance statement. The only solution would appear to be mandatory notification of the primary or secondary care trust regarding the existence of an advance statement by that individual—such mandatory notification raises issues of civil liberties.

The healthcare ethics problem is that of confidentiality. Professional guidance on ACP stipulates regarding advance care plans that 'Information cannot be shared with anyone, unless the individual concerned has agreed to disclosure.'[19] Patients' consent must be sought before such care plans are shared among health care professionals. This is of course because such plans are likely to contain very personal information. Consent to disclosure cannot be obtained once the patient is dead. So ideally from a moral perspective patients should be asked when they make or authorize their care plan/advance statement whether they are happy that it be shared with health care managers/clinical governance departments for the purposes of audit.

An educational paper on ethics in audit and research noted that many units rule that audit 'never involves disturbance of patients over and above normal clinical management. There is no extra data collection and no extra interventions or clinical assessments'. The author helpfully explained that moderate changes to clinical practice might need ethical review because the changes may be ineffective.[20] Ethical review of audit of the preferred place of care and death policy is arguably necessary and could be illuminating, but sadly is not even suggested!

It should be noted that the original Preferred Place of Care ACP document contained an intrinsic audit function—this document was withdrawn because of ethical and legal problems, not least with confidentiality. The audit function was abandoned when the new Preferred Priorities for Care document was designed. So we already have experience of the ethical (and legal) problems of audits regarding this goal of care.

8.2.v The role of family members

Family members and close friends are very often involved in the care of patients at the end of life, frequently taking a practical caring role and associated responsibility, even when outside professional help is provided. In some cases the location of care for the patient will have financial consequences for the spouse or partner of the patient, for example if a package of care at home, or care home placement, is required and is not funded via the NHS. So family members usually have completely legitimate interests and preferences of their own regarding the location of care for the patient.

By contrast, ACP and care planning is about eliciting and achieving the preferences of the patient. These preferences will usually be influenced by the availability, ability, and willingness of family members to adopt the caring role required. Very often patients and their family carers reach amicable agreement and the patient's expressed preference reflects that agreement. But inevitably conflicts and lesser differences of opinion arise between patients and other family members over this issue. Researchers in Canada found that half of patient/family caregiver dyads disagreed on preferred location of death.[21] Such conflicts are usually genuine and understandable conflicts of interest and are not due to what might be judged 'bad behaviour' or 'dysfunctional relationships' on either side.

For example, a patient with early dementia may make an advance care plan stating a wish to be cared for and to die at home. But if this is to be achieved, there will be a very major impact on a caring spouse or partner and/or grown-up children. The patient with dementia is likely to require 24 hours/day supervision for a period of months to years, plus physical care for an unpredictable period. The inevitable physical and mental tasks of caring can be very burdensome, even to the strongest and most loving of family members.

But if there is an imperative to achieve the patient's choice, then the interests of the family must be overridden if they conflict with the patient's preferences, even though the patient's choice often has a profound effect on the lives and wellbeing of family carers. Of course family members may become 'patients' themselves through a deterioration in their own physical or mental health; this adverse effect was noted in the family caregivers of patients with advanced chronic obstructive pulmonary disease.[22] But the extent to which the family's health needs should then be taken into account, and by whom, is unclear. There will be other situations where the patient will request residential care, inpatient specialist palliative care, or to remain in a familiar hospital ward, while family members have different preferences, including care at home.

It is a matter of ethical importance that decisions regarding the location of patients' care and death tend to have a greater impact on family members than do treatment decisions made by or on behalf of the patient. Treatment decisions affect what might be termed the bodily and mental integrity of the patient, but not that of the family. By contrast, location of care decisions can often affect the bodily and mental integrity of family members when they are caring for the patient at home. Anne-Marie Slowther, a clinical ethicist, noted the likely conflict of interests in an article on the role of the family in patient care. She commented that 'Various ethical conflicts may arise and consideration needs to be given to the autonomy and best interests of both patient and carer. . . . Caring for a patient in the social context of their family can create ethical difficulties that are not readily resolvable by reliance on principles alone.'[23]

The controversial ethical issue here is the extent to which the welfare and interests of family carers should be overridden by the preferences of patients regarding location of care and death. Readers will wish to consider whether it is ethically justifiable for professionals to support the patient's preference and strive to achieve it when it is clear that so doing is likely to result in significant physical or mental harms to family carers. We will return to this topic in Section 10.3 on the interests of relatives.

8.2.vi **Use of resources**

In a publicly funded health care service such as the NHS the values of equity in distribution of resources, and of cost-effectiveness to ensure best use of resources, are generally understood and agreed to be important. Thus the *End of life care strategy* lists as its aims 'choice, quality, equality and value for money.'

The ethical question then arises regarding what happens to the values of equity, cost-effectiveness, and providing care of an adequate quality if there is a strong or overriding imperative to achieve patients' choices in terms of place of care and death? In the event of a conflict between these values, for example if achieving a patient's choice is neither equitable nor cost-effective, is it then ethically justifiable not to achieve the patient's choice?

We shall consider initially the value of provision of care of adequate quality, which we abbreviate to the value 'quality'. At first sight it may appear that this value cannot be compromised, and that an adequate quality of care must be provided wherever the patient is cared for. But the ethical situation is not so simple, as the following example shows.

Patients who are in their own homes, and who have capacity to make the decision regarding location of care, can decide to remain at home (assuming they are not manifesting mental disorders which would warrant detention elsewhere under the Mental Health Act). But providing an adequate quality of care at home may not be feasible, perhaps because of manpower constraints (especially if continuous 24-hour care is needed for a prolonged period), or if there are safety issues for professional carers such as an aggressive dog or hoarding behaviour such that the extremely cluttered home environment prevents safe lifting equipment from being used.

So situations will arise in which it will not be possible to achieve both the patient's preference for place of care and death and the value of adequate quality of care. If the patient is entitled to be at, and decides to be at, the location where the value 'quality' cannot be achieved, then the quality of care provided might justifiably be compromised. In the example above it is clear that there cannot be a duty to provide a very large package of care at home if the manpower in the community simply is not available to do so. Nor would it be justifiable to put the health and safety of staff at significant risk in order to achieve an adequate quality of care in the location of the patient's choice.

Perhaps the most frequent conflicts of values are between achieving the patient's choice in place of care and death, and the values of both equity and cost-effectiveness. Care arrangements which consume large amounts of money, manpower or both are ethically problematic because they necessarily entail opportunity costs for other patients in a system where resources are limited. Equity requires that limited resources are distributed as fairly as possible, but this may not be compatible with achieving choices for every patient.

For example, it is often the case that community manpower resources are limited for hands-on practical nursing care tasks, especially over long holiday weekends and school holidays when carers may be less available. The situation could arise where three patients in an acute hospital who live in the same area all wish to go home, and all are in need of end of life care. But manpower resources are limited. If one patient's needs require a very large package of care, providing it might mean that neither of the other two can have adequate care provided at home so their discharge will be delayed, possibly resulting in their death in hospital rather than at home. Alternatively, one can argue that the two with moderate care needs should be discharged using the available community resources, but the third (who requires the largest care package) would then remain in hospital, possibly resulting in death in hospital.

In real life the situation is more complex than this in terms of equitable distribution of resources. The resources for end of life care are frequently not 'ring-fenced'. So patients in need of care in the last months of their lives are competing for resources with patients who have very different needs, such as ongoing care for disability due to chronic disease. The question then is: to what extent is it justifiable that the aim of achieving the patient's preferred place of care and death should compromise the provision of care to patients equally dependent on care but not currently approaching death? Should the fact that patients are approaching the end of their lives give them a greater entitlement to a limited resource than those who are not at the end of their lives?

Obviously other clinical factors are relevant, such as whether a patient is stable enough to wait a certain length of time for care to be available in the preferred place. But the basic ethical question is whether a patient's preference for place of care/death, in the context of end of life care, should necessarily trump the preferences for location of care for other patients (either terminally ill or not) given that limitations of resources render it impossible to achieve the preferences of all. This is summarized by asking whether achieving this choice for end of life care patients can justifiably trump the value called equity.

Readers might object that the answer to the choice/equity conflict is to increase the desired resources of manpower and money so that achieving patients' preferences for place of care and death does not compromise care to other patients. But then one runs into the problems of satisfying the ethical requirement for cost-effectiveness in a publicly funded system.

We noted in discussion of resource constraints in Section 4.1 that NICE decided to change its policy so as to raise its nominal cost-effectiveness limit for life-prolonging treatment (£30,000 per quality-adjusted life year (QALY)), just for patients at the end of life. This decision overturned their previous (and much more defensible) policy of applying the cost-effectiveness threshold equally to all patients. The ethical arguments (and controversy) about cost-effectiveness thresholds would obviously apply to resource expenditure on place of care/death in end of life care. Is being cared for in the location of your choice more highly valued at the end of life than outside that context? Should more than £30,000 per QALY, perhaps even as much as £70,000 per QALY, be spent to achieve the preferred place of care and death? Moreover, are the opportunity costs to other non-end-of-life patients justified? We leave readers to reach their own conclusions on what ought to be national policy on this issue.

If the surveys of the public cited in the *End of life care strategy* are correct, the following evidence will greatly influence the costs of care:

[A] Most people would prefer to be cared for at home, as long as high quality care can be assured and as long as they do not place too great a burden on their families and carers;

[B] Some research has shown that some people (particularly older people) who live alone wish to live at home for as long as possible, although they wish to die elsewhere where they can be certain not to be on their own;

[C] Some people on the other hand would not wish to be cared for at home, because they do not want family members to have to care for them. Many of these patients would prefer to be cared for in a hospice;

[D] Most, but not all, people would prefer not to die in a hospital—although this is in fact where most people do die. [24]

Achieving patients' preferences for place of care and death will mean having the resources to enable patients to be at home (sometimes with a very large package of care or 24-hour continuous 1:1 care). This is needed for groups A and B. Group B patients will also need somewhere to be cared for at the time of their death which is not home, so they will require nursing home or specialist palliative care or hospital inpatient care. Group C patients will require mainly hospice/specialist palliative care beds. Group D comprises a minority of patients who want to die in hospital, so appropriate inpatient hospital care will be needed. Three points should be made with reference to meeting the preferences of these groups of patients.

First, it cannot be assumed that care at home for patients who are frail and living alone, or are very dependent, or whose families are unwilling or unable to provide some care, will actually consume less resources than residential care in a rest or nursing home. It may consume more resources in terms of both manpower and money. A pilot programme by the charity Marie Curie Cancer Care to try to enable terminally ill cancer patients to die at home found that the costs of care for the last 8 weeks of life were similar for the intervention group (of whom 42% died at home) as for the control group (of whom 19% died at home).[25] But this does not mean that care at home for all patients would cost the same or less than residential care or current usual care. The resource consequences of care at home for that majority of patients who currently die in hospital or care homes are not known but could be estimated; it is possible that those costs at home could be significantly greater. When patients are very close to death (approximately within the last 3 months so far as this can be foreseen) the costs of their care are currently met by the NHS via 'continuing healthcare funding' arrangements. The financial and manpower costs of 24-hour continuous 1:1 care at home for this period, especially if two carers are needed at intervals for transfers between bed and chair, will be extremely high.

Second, patients who are dying in hospital and not at their preferred location for death require transfer to that location quickly, and certainly before their condition deteriorates to the point where the journey would be distressing and deleterious for them. If their preferred location for death is home, then a (possibly large) package of hands-on care must be available at home almost immediately in order to achieve their preference. In addition, patients already at home may rapidly become much less well, requiring frequent or continuous hands-on care within a matter of hours. In order to make all this care available within hours there would have to be not just adequate but spare resource capacity in the community. But maintaining spare capacity is expensive, and is not normally condoned in the NHS as it is judged not cost-effective. Similar problems arise when the preferred location is a nursing home near home—spare nursing home capacity is needed to achieve prompt placement. We have already noted in Chapter 1 that consumer choice requires spare capacity, and this is but one example.

The third issue relates to costs and cost-effectiveness. If the available evidence is correct, about 25% of patients (groups B and C mainly) would prefer to die in hospice/specialist palliative care beds, but the resource of these beds can accommodate only about 5% of patients who die (see Section 8.2.ii). So if the writers of national strategy are committed to achieving patients' preferences for place of death, the availability of these beds will have to be considerably increased. The Strategy expresses no such aim. If the number of hospice/

specialist palliative care beds was to be at least quadrupled, and if such beds were to be funded by the NHS as part of a commitment to patient choice, then the resource consequences would be great: the costs of specialist palliative care beds to the NHS would rise from its current level of £34 million to £996 million, according to the data from the *End of life care strategy*.[26]

Inpatient specialist palliative care and acute hospital care are both expensive. They are expensive because of the nature of care they are set up to provide. If their use is to be cost-effective, then ideally patients in those beds should be those who actually require the facilities and staff:patient ratios which specialist palliative care and hospitals rightly provide.

The 2004 NICE guidance on *Improving supportive and palliative care for adults with cancer* stipulated that the patients in receipt of the scarce resources of specialist palliative care should be those with 'complex problems', which generalist services in hospitals or the community cannot deal with effectively.[27] Complex problems are defined as:

> those that affect multiple domains of need and are severe and intractable, involving a combination of difficulties in controlling physical and/or psychological symptoms, the presence of family distress and social and/or spiritual problems. They also exceed the capacity and competence of providers to meet the needs and expectations of the patient and carers.

NICE quite reasonably set out to allocate the scarce resource of specialist palliative care according to patient need, not according to patient choice. If instead, in order to achieve patients' preferred place of care and death, inpatient specialist palliative care were to be allocated according to patient choice, three serious adverse consequences would ensue. The first is that many patients would be disappointed and disillusioned; current evidence indicates that these scarce beds can accommodate only about one in five of the patients who would choose to be there, so four out of five of those patients would be disappointed. The second is that patients not able to make a choice (because of lack of capacity and lack of an advance statement indicating an advance choice) would not be able to gain access to these beds, because they would all be occupied by those who had expressed their choice for one of those beds, either contemporaneously or in an advance statement. The third, and ethically the most serious consequence, is that those patients who really did have complex problems that could not be resolved outside of the specialist environment would only rarely gain access to specialist beds, because they would be occupied by patients who chose to be cared for and die in the specialist environment.

The same sorts of argument apply to the use of hospital beds for that minority of patients who would choose to die there. Acute hospital beds, especially those on oncology wards, are very often in short supply. If they are to be allocated according to patient preference rather than according to patients' need for the services they provide, then it is possible that patients who do need an acute hospital bed might be denied it.

It is obvious that if a patient's care and treatment needs do not necessitate a specialist palliative care bed or an acute hospital bed, both of which are high-cost, then it is not cost-effective to accommodate the patient in those locations. By contrast, residential care would be cost-effective, provided of course that it could meet the patient's care needs. It has been argued that resources should be diverted from hospitals to the community to fund care at home,[28] but the funds released would not necessarily cover the costs of care for highly dependent patients at home. The consequences of actually closing the relevant hospital beds to release the resources must also be considered.

There is evidence indicating that 18% of patients aged over 85 years were in care homes in 2001, the main reasons for admission being physical dependence (associated with dementia and stroke in particular). Admission to a care home is considered the best option for many following comprehensive geriatric assessment.[29] This percentage is coherent with that of 17% of deaths occurring in care homes quoted by *End of life care strategy*.[30] What is not clear is whether these patients would have preferred care at home. The costs of their care at home could be very great, particularly where the cause of death is dementia.[31] If the policy of care and death in the place of the patient's choice is really to be implemented notwithstanding the costs, then these patients too must be cared for in their own homes if that is their choice. However, the high cost of care in their own homes would probably entail significant opportunity costs for other patients—issues of cost-effectiveness would arise which do not appear to have been considered.

These arguments together demonstrate that there are major ethical problems with the promotion of patient choice for place of care/death as a value which overrides the values of equity and cost-effectiveness.

We have discussed the issue of preferred place of care and death in detail because it is now a major issue, both professionally and politically, in end of life care. We leave readers to work out for themselves how the inevitable conflicts between the value of choice and the values of equity, cost-effectiveness and sometimes quality should be resolved. It does appear to be very difficult to justify allowing the value of choice to 'trump' the values of equity and cost-effectiveness, and perhaps also quality of care. If preferred place of death is introduced as a performance measure, professionals must consider how to respond. The general practitioner Iona Heath has pointed out that when we are faced with a command from an authority it is our responsibility to judge whether the command is moral or immoral. She notes that it is our decision whether to obey a command, so long as we are not physically prevented from making that choice.[32] The problem in the NHS is that if we do not achieve well on a performance measure it may be our patients who are penalized.

8.3 ACP and preferred place of care and death: should we be asking a different question?

The *End of life care strategy* makes reference to large scale surveys of the public to ascertain people's preferences and priorities in relation to end of life care.[33] But it does not comment on what was important to people other than place of care, a high quality of care if they are at home (in order to minimize burdens on the family), and not being alone at death. So we do not appear to know from large surveys what other aspects of care at the end of life are important to people.

In Section 7.7 we note that the limited evidence on ACP indicates that people preferred goal- or outcome-orientated advance statements. The Joint guidance group who searched the evidence base did not report which individual factors patients considered most important. Furthermore, there is very little evidence from the UK. At the time of writing, there are no published findings from the pilot study of the Preferred Priorities for Care document which contains a general question about preferences and priorities for future care.

It seems strange to have singled out the issue of place of care and death, with the implication that it is the most important issue for patients, or at least extremely important. Perhaps other factors such as the quality of care and symptom control, and having family present as desired, would also be important to patients. It is possible that the issue of place of death has been singled out simply because it is (relatively) easy to use as an outcome/performance measure.

Whatever the reason for attributing so much importance to place of death, it does seem a rather belittling view of human nature to assume that it is the most important factor for people facing the end of life. Is where they die really the most important issue about death for most people? We do not seem to know, and as a hypothesis it actually sounds rather implausible. Readers might like to reflect on patients they have known and friends and family of their own who have died—was location of death the most important thing to them? Or was it having loved ones close, being free from pain, not being a burden on others?

The presence of the specific question regarding place of care in the two nationally recommended documents is actually directing patients to consider this one issue. It might be better to ask only a single open question about preferences, such as 'what would be important to you as you approach the end of your life?' The answers to such a question would then truly represent the patients' priorities—not organizational, or professional, or political priorities! If ACP is really about the patient's priorities, documents should be designed to elicit precisely those.

8.4 **Conclusions**

1) Advance care planning policy instructs professionals to ask patients about their preferred place of care and death.

2) Attempts to achieve patients' previously stated preferences on this matter may not always be in their best interests in the later situation when they have lost capacity; making decisions on the basis of their 'best interests' is a legal requirement of the Mental Capacity Act.

3) Patients' preferences may also conflict with those of the family, and will certainly consume as-yet-unquantified resources.

4) More important, it may be argued that ACP as a whole is asking the wrong question, or is omitting several questions which may be important to patients, or that it should ask only a single open question about what is important to the patient.

5) Singling out the patients' preferences for place of care and death may simply be a process to establish an outcome or performance measure which is quantifiable and easy to audit.

References

1. World Health Organization (2004). *Palliative care: the solid facts*. WHO, Geneva, p. 17.
2. National Institute for Clinical Excellence (2004). *Improving supportive and palliative care for adults with cancer*. NICE, London, p. 118.
3. Department of Health (2008). *End of life care strategy*. DoH, London, p. 27.
4. Department of Health, op. cit. (ref. 3), p. 33.
5. Mayor S (2008). End of life strategy offers home based nursing care 24 hours a day for dying patients. *BMJ* **337**:a871.
6. South West Strategic Health Authority (2008). *The strategic framework for improving health in the South West 2008/9 to 2010/11*. South West Strategic Health Authority, Taunton, pp. 77–78. Summary version, p. 18.
7. Riley J (2008). A strategy for end of life care in the UK. *BMJ* **337**:a943.
8. Riley J, Smith C, Thick M (2008). Experience from the Royal Marsden. *BMJ* **337**:a2290.
9. Hughes N (2008). Clinical dashboards and open kimonos. *BMJ* **337**:a787.
10. Department of Health, op. cit. (ref. 3), p. 27.
11. Higginson IJ (2003). *Priorities and preferences for end of life care in England, Wales and Scotland*. Cicely Saunders Foundation, Scottish Partnership for Palliative Care and National Council for Hospice and Specialist Palliative Care, London.

12. Wade DT (2005). Ethics, audit and research: all shades of grey. *BMJ* **330**:468–73.

13. Gomes B, Higginson IJ (2008). Where people die (1974–2030): past trends, future projections and implications for care. *Palliative Medicine* **22**:33–41.

14. Department of Health, op. cit. (ref. 3), p. 27.

15. Bevan G, Hood C (2006). Have targets improved performance in the English NHS? *BMJ* **332**:419–22.

16. Thomson-Moore A (2008). Doctors' infantalisation. *BMJ* **337**:a791.

17. Rawlinson N (2008). Harms of target driven care. *BMJ* **337**:a195.

18. Department for Constitutional Affairs (2007). Mental Capacity Act 2005. Code of Practice. The Stationery Office, Norwich, p. 81.

19. End of Life Care Programme (2008). *Advance care planning: a guide for health and social care staff.* Available at http://www.endoflifecareforadults.nhs.uk/eolc/ppc.htm (accessed on 16.1.09).

20. Wade D, op. cit. (ref. 12), p. 469.

21. Stajduhar KI, Allan DE, Cohen SR, Heyland DK (2008). Preferences for location of death of seriously ill hospitalised patients: perspectives from Canadian patients and their family caregivers. *Palliative Medicine* **22**:85–88.

22. Simpson AC, Rocker MR (2008). Advanced chronic obstructive pulmonary disease: impact on informal caregivers. *Journal of Palliative Care* **24**:49–54.

23. Slowther A (2006). The role of the family in patient care. *Clinical Ethics* **1**:191–3.

24. Department of Health, op. cit. (ref. 3), p. 27–8.

25. Addicott R, Dewar S (2008). *Improving choice at the end of life.* King's Fund, London, p. 10.

26. Department of Health, op. cit. (ref. 3), p. 151.

27. NICE, op. cit. (ref. 2), p. 122.

28. National Audit Office (2008). *End of life care.* The Stationery Office, Norwich, p. 7.

29. Burns E, Cracknell A (2007). When should older people go into care? *Clin Med* **7**:508–511.

30. Department of Health, op. cit. (ref. 3), p. 26.

31. Dartington T (2008). Dying from dementia—a patient's journey. *BMJ* **337**:a1712.

32. Heath I (2008). Dare to use your own intelligence. *BMJ* **337**:a1319.

33. Department of Health, op. cit. (ref. 3), p. 27.

Choice, assisted suicide and euthanasia

In two Western countries (Belgium and The Netherlands) voluntary euthanasia has been legalized, and physician-assisted suicide (PAS) has been legalized in The Netherlands and in the state of Oregon, USA. In Switzerland it is lawful for anyone to assist another person to commit suicide, provided that the motive is entirely honourable.[1] In the UK and other countries there is ongoing debate about whether assisted suicide and/or voluntary euthanasia should be legalized. We should note that there is a distinction between laws which permit anyone to assist suicide, and those which permit only physicians to assist suicide.

Curiously, many of those most opposed to the legalizing of assisted suicide or voluntary euthanasia are also very much in favour of patient choice. Those opposed to such legalization would include the majority of doctors surveyed in 2006 by the UK Royal College of Physicians,[2] and by the BMA,[3] the majority of European doctors surveyed, with a larger majority opposed in the specialties of palliative medicine, geriatrics and oncology[4] and many politicians. But, given that choice is so highly valued, it is not immediately clear why the ideology of choice should not include the ultimate choice to receive assistance to end your own life, or indeed to have someone else deliberately kill you, at the time of your own choosing. In relation to our discussions in this book, if such a high value is placed on choice in end of life care, there is a requirement to justify restricting that choice by not permitting PAS and euthanasia.

In this chapter we shall criticize three common arguments in favour of assisted suicide and voluntary euthanasia: the argument from moral equivalence (in its various forms); the argument from the right to die; the argument from human dignity. To criticize these arguments is not of course to reject the case for PAS or assisted suicide or euthanasia. It is just to say that such a case should not depend on these three extremely weak or false arguments. The strongest case for PAS or assisted suicide is very simple and does not need to depend on fallacious reasoning. We shall outline this case at the end of the chapter and we shall leave it to readers to make up their own minds on this controversial and much-debated issue. But readers' views should not be determined by slogans, such as a 'right to die', and they should bear in mind the ultimate conclusions which some have reached via the 'moral equivalence' argument. Clearly, readers' views ought not to be determined by statements which are factually false, such as appear from time to time in the media.

9.1 **The argument from 'moral equivalence'**

We shall discuss this argument (or cluster of arguments) only briefly here because they are stated more fully in Chapter 3. The general form of these arguments is: 'Doing X is morally equivalent to doing Y. Therefore if X is thought to be permissible so should Y be.' For the purposes of our discussion, X is either withholding or withdrawing life-prolonging treatment, or administering sedation with a risk of hastening death. Y is either euthanasia or PAS.

The argument could be put as follows. It could be asserted that if withholding or withdrawing treatment (because the patient refuses it, or because it is not producing an overall health benefit) results in the patient's death, then this is morally equivalent to causing the death of the patient. Since causing the patient's death by withholding or withdrawing potentially life-prolonging treatment is permissible, so should causing death by euthanasia or by assisting the patient's suicide be permissible. Alternatively, it would be asserted that sedating the terminally ill patient ('terminal sedation') to the extent that death may be hastened is morally equivalent to causing death. Therefore, if administering such sedation is permitted, then so should supplying drugs with the intent of enabling the patient to cause his/her own death, or administering lethal drugs in euthanasia, be permitted. Put another way, if action X is not considered wrong and unlawful, and action Y is morally equivalent to action X, how can action Y be wrong or unlawful?

These arguments rest on the claims that withholding and withdrawing life-prolonging treatment, or administering sedation which may hasten death, are 'morally equivalent' to causing death by euthanasia and to assisting the patient to cause his/her own death. These sorts of argument are commonly used in support of legalization of euthanasia and PAS—we hold that they are based on fundamental confusions.

We discussed the confusions at some length in Section 3.3, but note here the additional point that they depend on the unclear expression 'moral equivalence'. The 'equivalence' seems to be that the alleged outcomes are the same— the patient dies. But an (alleged) equivalent *outcome* is not the same as *moral* equivalence. Moral equivalence would require two further conditions: an equivalent *intention* and equivalent *causality*. But in the case of withholding or withdrawing treatment the intention is to end a non-beneficial procedure and/or one which the patient is refusing, and in the case of sedation the intention is to ease suffering, whereas in the case of PAS or euthanasia the intention is to kill the patient. Moreover, there is no equivalent causality. The easiest way to show this is to use a common legal test for causality—the 'but for' test. In negligence cases the victim must show that 'but for' the defendant's negligent action the injury (or death) would not have occurred.[5] But in end of life cases it would not be possible to demonstrate that 'but for' the withholding or withdrawing of treatment, or the sedation, the patient would not have died, for the patient would have died of the illness in any case. Indeed, if the treatment were withheld or withdrawn from a healthy patient, or the sedation given to a healthy patient, death would not occur. Intention to cause death, and causality regarding death, are therefore both evidently absent in withholding/withdrawing life-prolonging treatment or providing sedation at the end of life, and hence there can be no moral equivalence to PAS, far less active euthanasia.

There are two general assumptions behind our rejection of these weak arguments. The first assumption is that the only justification for medical treatment is that it provides a health benefit. If it does not provide a health benefit it should be withheld or withdrawn. Of course, most treatments also cause harms in the form of undesirable adverse effects. More realistically, then, we should say that the only justification for medical treatment is that it provides more benefits than harms, sometimes phrased as 'net benefit'. Statements to this effect are found in the UK consensus professional guidance for doctors.[6,7] Hence, allowing patients to die of their illnesses (letting die) has to be permitted when the harms and risks of potentially life-prolonging treatment clearly outweigh its benefits. The second assumption is that society needs to maintain its prohibition against killing (murder) in order to protect its members. In order to achieve these two aims the law has to uphold a clear distinction between killing and letting die.

In law an act of killing is murder if one person *intended* to cause and *did cause* the death of another. It is universally prohibited and is severely punished. Thus a charge of murder would be brought against a doctor who intended to cause and did cause the death of a patient. On the other hand, a doctor who withholds or withdraws a life-prolonging treatment from a patient because it cannot now provide net benefit, or because the patient refuses the treatment, clearly does not intend the patient's death, but rather intends to remove a treatment which is non-beneficial and also possibly harmful, or which is not wanted by the patient. The doctor is considered to have allowed a foreseen death to occur from natural causes and is not charged with murder. In this situation letting the patient die is legally permitted. Furthermore, if the only justification for providing the treatment is absent, it follows logically that there is a legal obligation to withhold or withdraw the treatment. The British Medical Association (BMA) guidance thus advises that life-prolonging treatment which is refused by a patient with capacity, or which cannot provide net benefit to a patient lacking capacity, should 'ethically and legally, be withheld or withdrawn'.[8]

Similarly, if a patient is agitated or distressed at the end of life it would be considered good practice to offer sedation if other means of alleviating the distress have failed. Sedation sufficient to cause drowsiness or diminished consciousness may have the effect of decreasing mobility and fluid and food intake, and this *may* make death more likely, but the intent in offering such treatment is to relieve the patient's suffering, not to end the patient's life. Symptom control at the end of life is judged to be ethically acceptable, indeed ethically required, even if, in rare circumstances, it may be one factor contributing to slightly earlier death than might otherwise have occurred. We discussed this issue in Section 6.3.

We thus agree with the current consensus view that there is *no* 'moral equivalence' between withholding and withdrawing life-prolonging treatments (where the patient is refusing them or they cannot provide net benefit), or providing sedation to alleviate distress in the dying even though it may hasten death, and PAS or euthanasia. Therefore it is entirely reasonable that the law should distinguish between them. But having said this it is important to be aware of the conclusions which some proponents are drawing from the 'moral equivalence' argument, since those conclusions would have profound effects on health care and probably also on societal values.

In their book entitled *Easeful death*, philosopher Mary Warnock and doctor Elizabeth Macdonald use the 'moral equivalence' argument extensively in support of legalizing PAS and euthanasia. First, they refer to a patient's refusal of 'intrusive and distressing' palliative chemotherapy as having 'caused her own death'.[9] Second, they describe doctors withdrawing ventilation from a patient with capacity who was clearly refusing it as concerned that they 'should deliberately bring the life of the patient to an end.'[10] Third, they regard withholding or withdrawing life-prolonging treatment because further treatment is futile as 'non-voluntary euthanasia'.[11] They are thus arguing that in the first two cases there is moral equivalence to assisting a suicide and in the third (and possibly second) case moral equivalence to euthanasia. In other words, they are arguing that the doctors intended to cause and did in fact cause the death of the patients. Following the pattern of the argument we outlined above, they later reach the conclusion that if what is already legally permitted is morally equivalent to PAS and euthanasia, then PAS and euthanasia should be legalized. But there is no moral equivalence. In the first two cases the patients' (reasonable) decisions are to refuse intrusive, distressing and possibly ineffective treatments, and the doctors' decisions are to obey the law and accept these decisions. In the third case the medical decision is based on the best interests of the patient, since the treatment holds no prospect of benefit.

They develop their argument in an even more startling way. In relation to a person with dementia who has lost the ability to express wishes and feelings, they argue that 'We should in time be prepared to contemplate not merely allowing him to die by withholding treatment if he falls ill, but actually and compassionately causing his death.'[12] Thus they explicitly express support for non-voluntary euthanasia of the demented, and one of their fundamental grounds for this is the claim of 'moral equivalence' to current ethically and legally accepted practice.

The general public are frequently exposed to the 'moral equivalence' argument through the media, in support of PAS and euthanasia. A notable example of this was an article by Simon Jenkins in the *Guardian* newspaper in 2008.[13] He argued that currently two-thirds of deaths are caused by premeditated acts of 'killing' by doctors, asserting that one-third of deaths are caused by deliberate morphine overdose and one-third by removal of life support. He then asserted that since judges cannot realistically prosecute two-thirds of the medical profession (presumably for 'killing' their patients), they are 'on the verge of rewriting the law' so that PAS and euthanasia, also acts of killing, will be legalized. He is thus arguing that killing by doctors is already occurring for the majority of patients, and since it cannot be prosecuted it would be appropriate to legalize the morally equivalent forms of killing, i.e. PAS and euthanasia. This is an example of the moral equivalence argument, albeit rather bizarre, extreme, and inclusive of some statements unlikely to be substantiated as facts!

We have described the 'moral equivalence' argument in detail not merely to demonstrate why it should be regarded as implausible at the least, and false by philosophical and legal standards, but also to demonstrate that it apparently leads to conclusions which would be unacceptable even to staunch supporters of PAS and euthanasia.

9.2 **The argument from the 'right to die'**

The language of rights, including human rights, is prevalent in health care ethics and policy-making at the moment. Indeed, 'rights' seems to have replaced 'autonomy' as the 'must-use' term. Autonomy is a capacity which we have or do not have, or have to a limited extent, and it is from autonomy that (most) moral rights derive. We can infer from the capacity for autonomy possessed by all mature adults with broadly normal cognitive function that such autonomous adults have the (moral) right to act as they please, provided they are not harming others. This is the basic principle of liberal-democratic society. It would of course require to be modified in certain situations, such as in time of war, but we shall let it stand in this broad-brush picture, and consider whether there is a right to die, or even a human right to die.

9.2.i A right to die?

The question is commonly posed, but it is an odd question. It might be said that we do not need a *right* to die because we are all going to die anyway, whether we like it or not! Death, it might be said, is a natural occurrence with a causal explanation. The language of rights does not seem appropriate. Of course, what the expression may (sometimes) mean is a right to be *allowed to* die. This might be said in a context in which a patient wishes to discontinue life-prolonging treatment. But such a right already exists—the right to withhold or withdraw consent to treatment. Even life-prolonging treatment may legally be refused, although doctors sometimes have anxieties about possible legal repercussions from withholding or withdrawing life-prolonging treatment, and some may also have moral scruples. None the less, such a right exists.

The right to refuse treatment is not the same, however, as the right to be actively assisted in causing one's own death, or the right to have one's death deliberately caused by another. These latter rights (if they existed or could be brought into existence by legislation) would be rights against someone who would then have a correlative duty to assist. But such a right does not now exist in the UK, although it does in a very small number of jurisdictions, such as The Netherlands. Is it morally persuasive to argue that such a right should be created and put on the statute book? To clarify this question and consider possible answers to it we shall provide a brief account of some conceptual distinctions in the theory of rights.

Rights are necessarily correlated with duties (although there are contexts in which duties can exist where there are no correlative rights—for example, a duty not to destroy wild flowers). What are the duties correlative with this broad liberal principle of rights, and who has these duties? The answer is that we all have duties not to interfere without consent in another person's right to act at pleasure, unless of course that action is harming others. Normally, of course, we do what we choose, without thinking of rights. For example, I might walk to the car park whistling, glad to be going home after a heavy day. I would not assert that I had a right to do so unless I were challenged, for example by the Chief Executive. We might call such rights 'rights of action' or 'freedoms', and note that they are constituted by the (normally unchallenged) moral rules underpinning our everyday action.

However, there is another type of right which we might call a 'right of recipience' or a 'claim'. In the case of such rights the correlative duties are owed by specific persons or groups. For example, if I borrow your book you have a right of recipience against me to have it returned and I have a duty to ensure that it is returned to you. Rights of recipience arise from undertakings, and the undertakings involve the use of the conventions of an accepted social practice or institution. For example, the practice of lending and borrowing is widely accepted in our society and the practice is constituted by certain conventions. These of course vary from the informal conventions of book-lending to the formal conventions of mortgages. But the basic principle of reciprocal rights and duties remains the same.

Before we apply these distinctions to the choice agenda as it affects assisted suicide and euthanasia we should note two further conceptual points about rights. First, since rights and duties are correlative, a right can exist only when a duty is possible. Second, it is well known that duties can conflict, but so also can rights. Dr A's wife and family may have a right to his time, and Dr A's hospital trust may also have a right to his skills. Dr A may therefore at times be faced with these and other conflicting rights and therefore not always be sure where his duty lies.

How do these distinctions apply to the alleged right to assisted suicide or voluntary euthanasia? A right to assisted suicide or euthanasia would be a right of recipience. A right to be *allowed* to commit suicide already exists as a right of action or a freedom, in the sense that it is not legally an offence to do so. But it follows from the very term 'assisted' that another person is involved. Hence, a right to assisted suicide must be a right of recipience—a right against someone who thereby acquires a duty to assist. A right to euthanasia necessarily entails a right against someone who thereby acquires a duty to administer the lethal means. But who should be the person who acquires the duty in each case?

The usual answer is that it should be the doctor. Indeed, it is often assumed that it must be the doctor. But this assumption must be questioned. Here we must remember the two points we noted about rights—that it must be possible for them to be exercised, or that the correlative duty must be feasible; and that rights, like duties, can conflict.

As far as the first point goes it would be easily possible (in the practical sense) to exercise the right to assisted suicide and/or euthanasia because there is nothing technically (as distinct from morally) difficult about the exercise of the duties, that is of assisting suicide or killing someone with a lethal injection.

One could not reasonably claim that assisting suicide or administering a lethal medication requires medical training, although some knowledge of what lethal dose to prescribe, and how to administer the injection, would be necessary. It follows that while doctors or nurses could do it, so could many others who do not have their extensive training. For example, it could be a job for journalists between big stories, or MPs who have lost their seats, or unemployed philosophers.

And the fact that, technically, assisted suicide and euthanasia could be provided by non-doctors has a bearing on the second point about rights—that rights can conflict. Doctors traditionally have duties of care towards their patients and patients have correlative rights to expect certain standards of care, and (despite the effects of political interference) they still do for the most part trust their doctors and professional staff. It is arguable that an inner tension would be created in the duty of care if it were to include a duty to assist with the suicide of a patient, or more starkly in the case of voluntary euthanasia, a duty to kill the patient. Moreover, those in palliative care maintain that there is also a duty of care to families. It is not necessary to take this duty to the lengths it is taken in specialist palliative care to agree that families are likely to be anxious or distressed if their doctor is also the one who assists in the killing or the suicide of their loved one.

From the patient's point of view it should be remembered that a right may (ethically) be exercised only if it is not harming others. It is notorious that a suicide in the family is psychologically disturbing and may engender feelings of guilt in the survivors. It is known that patients often perceive themselves to be a burden and families may feel guilt if patients resort to PAS or euthanasia partly for this reason.[14] Of course, psychological disturbances happen in families, but perhaps it is not for the law to create another possibility for such disturbance. And there is another perhaps more important side to the family issues. As we live longer we shall certainly be spending more of the family inheritance, and we may unwittingly impose a burden of care on our loved ones. A temptation might then be brought into existence to put some pressure on the frail elderly to move prematurely to the exit. We shall return to this argument later in Section 9.4.

More significant than the possible harm to the family there is the harm to society. There are two aspects to this, one which is broad and cultural and the other which is down-to-earth and practical. The broad and cultural issue is of importance for it concerns the sort of society in which we wish to live. Do we wish to live in a society in which a belief in the sanctity of life, as something which should not be taken, is maintained? Do we wish to live in a society in which we actually try to prevent suicide?[15] Legalizing assisted suicide or voluntary euthanasia will not destroy this belief in the sanctity of life and in the prohibition against killing, but it may over time begin to weaken it.

The down-to-earth and practical aspect concerns the premises which might be used for assisting suicide. Experience in Switzerland suggests that the public do not welcome the presence of an institution for PAS in their backyard, and the death tourism it may bring with it.[16] Leaving aside the black humour of the bodies going down the stairs we are taken back again to the culture of a society which sanctions such activities.

9.2.ii **Human rights and the 'right to die'**

It might be argued that we have not considered the claim that there is a special sort of 'right to die'—a human right. On the face of it, to claim that the human right to life can give rise to a human right to die does not seem very plausible. The human right to life was introduced to try to protect those who are mouldering in jails in tyrannous regimes, awaiting execution for, say, distributing a leaflet. To such victims it would seem a bitter irony that the right to life, which is being denied to them, is being used as a ground for alleging a right to assisted suicide or euthanasia. It would be extreme black humour to say that these victims, whose right to life has been denied, are about to have an 'assisted death'. Nevertheless, there have been several attempts to derive a human right to assisted death from the human right to life. We shall discuss just one such attempt, which we take from an editorial in the *BMJ*:

> Every human rights convention recognises a fundamental right to life. Paradoxically as it might at first seem, this entails a right to die also. For life in the phrase "the right to life" does not mean bare existence; it means existence that has a certain minimum quality for its possessors, where the minimum is quite rich, giving its possessors access to a range of basic human goods such as relationships, and in which they are as free as reasonably possible from distress and pain.
>
> The idea that the right to life is a right to life of a certain minimum quality implies that mere existence is not an automatic good . . . . When individuals maturely judge that their quality of life is below the minimum, they have the right to die if they have a settled and reasoned wish to do so. Considerations of humanity then further imply that they have a supplementary right to assistance of the kind that medical science can provide in dying painlessly and easily, since this concerns the quality of the lived experience of dying.[17]

This argument has three steps:

1) The (human) right to life is not just to bare existence, rather it is to a life with a certain quality.

2) When that quality falls below a certain minimum, the human beings acquire a right to die.

3) Common humanity implies that they acquire a further right to assisted death by medical science.

All three steps are highly questionable. The human right to life has never been understood to be a right to a life with a good quality, however desirable such a life might be. The right to life is what is sometimes called a negative right— a right not to be arbitrarily killed. Second, it does not *follow* from the first premise that when people's lives fall below a certain quality they then acquire a right to die. They might acquire a social or economic right to support or to *health care* (if we use the humanitarian argument), but it is not clear why we are forced by logic to say they acquire a right to die. Finally, to say that humanitarian considerations 'imply' a further right to be assisted in dying, i.e. that doctors have a duty to assist in suicide, or to perform euthanasia, is simply spurious logic, a misleading use of the logical term 'imply'. The question is whether it could ever be a part of a doctor's duty to assist with suicide or perform euthanasia. That is a difficult question of morality and public policy and the answer to it cannot be derived by invalid logic from false premises.

The language of rights has been used extensively in arguments about legalizing PAS and euthanasia, but where those arguments are clearly false (as in the immediately preceding analysis) they should not be influential. Two further examples demonstrate how the language of rights is being invoked in this debate to support PAS and euthanasia, with controversial results!

The first is from Jenkins' article in the *Guardian*. He wrote: 'There cannot be a human freedom so personal as ordering the circumstances of one's death. Yet Britain is instinctively collectivist, enveloped in prejudice, religion, taboo and prohibition. We are told how to die by the state, with no consideration for individual choice.'[18] He is asserting that there is a 'human freedom' to 'order' the circumstances of one's death, but what he is speaking of is obviously not a freedom to act without interference. Instead, it is a right of recipience that someone else will have the duty to assist you in your choice, simply on the grounds that it is your choice. He is asserting an almost tyrannical notion of the right to choice, which would inescapably impose the duty on others to enable you to achieve your choice. In examples such as this, language is being used in such a way as to produce spurious arguments very loosely based on the idea of human rights.

The second example is a chain of argument from Warnock and Macdonald in their book *Easeful death*. In relation to patients being allowed to die of their illness, they state that 'It is highly desirable that society . . . should think clearly about whether a patient should be legally entitled to decide to die'.[19] But it is clear that patients are already entitled to refuse life-prolonging treatment, so a change in the law is not required to achieve this end. These authors later suggest that there may be a 'natural' or 'human right' to choose to die, by which they actually mean a right of recipience such that, as they put it, people who autonomously want to die 'should have the acknowledged right to be helped to die.'[20] Not surprisingly they state that in such situations it is a doctor's duty to end the patient's life: 'In moral theory the doctor's duty taken to its logical conclusion requires him to do his utmost to follow patients' wishes and relieve their symptoms even if this requires the active (properly consented and monitored) termination of a patient's life.'[21] This sentence is a good example of rhetoric rather than rational argument. First, the use of the term 'moral theory' is intended to suggest a philosophical foundation for the claim, whereas all that is initially claimed is the truism that the doctor's duty is to relieve the patient's symptoms. Second, the expression 'taken to its logical conclusion' is intended to suggest that the conclusion cannot be denied without illogicality. But the conclusion does not *follow* logically; it is simply a re-assertion of the point at issue—whether it could ever be a doctor's duty to intend to kill a patient, granted that the first principle of all medical codes of ethics is 'First do no harm.'

The foregoing paragraph illustrates how rights language is being used to try to establish a right to PAS and euthanasia, with the correlative duty to assist in suicide or perform euthanasia being placed firmly and unequivocally on doctors.

The assertion of such a right plus the correlative duty has caused doctors to be concerned that conscientious objection to performing PAS and euthanasia would not be permitted if these practices were legalized—this reasonable concern was expressed by John Saunders, writing as chairman of the Royal College of Physicians committee on ethical issues in medicine.[22,23] Julian Savulescu, an ethicist in health care, has argued against allowing conscientious objection, stating that 'doctors who compromise the delivery of medical services to patients on conscience grounds must be punished through removal of licence to practise and other legal mechanisms'.[24] PAS and euthanasia, once seen as a right for patients via the health service, would inevitably be seen as a 'medical service'. Not surprisingly, Savulesco's views generated strong counter-argument![25]

There may be other arguments from human rights, but it does seem like an inhumane distortion of human rights to use them as grounds for assisting suicide or carrying out euthanasia, or for the legalization of these actions. Readers interested in the issues raised by patient rights in a publicly funded health service might wish to read a useful summary.[26]

How conclusive one way or another are the many arguments which can be assembled under the 'right to die' heading? We hope we have shown at the very least that the 'right to die' slogan is not clear, that some of the arguments put forward under that banner are false, and that overall the arguments for creating a right to PAS or voluntary euthanasia are extremely weak and definitely not conclusive one way or the other.

9.3 The argument from dignity

The argument from dignity to PAS or euthanasia can take several forms because the concept of dignity is complex. Within the UK, in a national report on dignity in care (including end of life care) for older people, the Healthcare Commission stated that 'Dignity is a human rights issue and should be the underlying principle for delivery of services.'[27] While admitting that no standard working definition of dignity exists, they quoted instead a statement by the charity Help the Aged which describes how a sense of dignity could be promoted: 'The use of appropriate forms of address, listening, and giving people choice, including them, respecting their need for privacy and politeness, and making them feel valued emerged as significant ways to maintain older people's sense of self-worth and dignity.'[28] So once again, choice and taking account of people's wishes is seen as central to maintenance of dignity. How should dignity be analysed?

9.3.i The analysis of dignity

When some aspect of human nature is threatened, people reach for one of a range of concepts to defend themselves. Sometimes it is 'freedom', sometimes it is 'human rights', and sometimes it is 'dignity'. We are suggesting then that 'dignity' does not name a property which human beings have, but rather it is a moral term suggesting how human beings should or should not be treated in a given social or individual context. This is why groups such as Help the Aged and the Healthcare Commission focus on how patients should be treated, rather than on trying to define or describe a property called 'dignity'.

As noted in the *Oxford textbook of palliative medicine*, '"dignity" in the dying process is a critical goal of palliative care . . . [but] there is little empirical research on how this term has been used by patients who are nearing death'.[29] Perhaps it is possible to be a little more precise than this implies, although such precision cannot be derived from empirical studies which authors such as Dr Chochinov have conducted. He concludes that individuals are likely to ascribe their own meaning or importance to the notion of dying with dignity; his work describes how clinicians may try to conserve that individual notion of dignity for patients.[30] In Arthur Frank's words, dignity (or indignity) claims must 'stand on' something.[31] Can we locate a foundation?

Here we might adapt and extend Daryl Pullman's term 'basic dignity'[32] which may be said to rest on basic human nature. Our contention is that dignity or indignity claims arise when some of the many aspects of basic human nature are being neglected or abused. For Kant the basis of human nature is its autonomy. This is understandable in his eighteenth-century century historical context in which human beings were emerging from a hierarchical type of society and moving towards a more egalitarian type of society with political democracy as a ruling idea. But although Kant's conception of basic human nature is sparse or minimal, it can still ground a large number of dignity or indignity claims relevant to end of life care and more generally. For example, granted that people are rational, self-determining and self-governing, it will be an affront to their dignity to lie to them, to delude them, to fail to consult them, to fail to go along with their *refusal* of life-prolonging treatment, or to contrive to find some way round their advance refusal of treatment.

But there are many other aspects of basic human nature as well as rationality. Human beings are mind–body unities; they are sentient as well as rational. Human beings have a strong dislike of physical pain, they have a desire to cover their bodies, especially their genital areas, and a desire for privacy when engaged in various bodily functions. Whether these desires are universal or simply enormously widespread is a question we can leave to one side. Certainly they extend well beyond Western civilization. It will follow from these widespread human desires that patients waiting in public places for clinicians to see them and clad only in inadequate gowns may well claim that their dignity has been violated, or patients who are not brought bedpans in good time may similarly feel that they have been degraded. Paradigmatically, patients who are left in 'total pain', like Ivan Illich in Tolstoy's story, are robbed of their dignity.[33]

This side of basic human nature is of course important in end of life care and it is one of the areas in which nurses have an important role. It is also interesting that the importance of this side of basic human nature increases as the patient's capacity for self-determination decreases. The majority of patients in end of life care will be very sick, and at some time lack capacity. Yet conceptions of dignified or undignified treatment still apply to them when they are semi-conscious or comatose. Indeed, the idea of 'basic human nature' as a ground for claims of dignity or indignity still apply to a dead body. This is a deeply rooted human idea which can be found at the centre of Sophocles' play *Antigone*. Creon, the ruler of a city state, has decreed that the body of Polyneices should be left outside the city walls to be eaten by vultures. Polyneices' sister, Antigone, argues with Creon, to the effect that there is a higher law, a law of nature, that we can all recognize, which insists that even the dead should be treated with dignity.[34]

Whereas it is reasonably easy to see what constitutes respect for dignity when we are dealing with the rational aspects of human nature (e.g. truth-telling and consent) and also for the bodily function aspects (pain relief and privacy mainly), it is less easy to know what will be considered a dignified treatment of a dead body. Here we can go back to Pullman's distinction between 'basic dignity' and 'personal dignity', the latter being subjective or peculiar to that individual.[35] Perhaps this idea of 'personal dignity' needs to broadened, for much that may appear 'personal' is likely to be cultural. This will apply especially to the treatment of a body after death, but may also apply to how a patient is examined and by whom. Again, some patients find having to be washed, and more generally the loss of physical independence, undignified. Hence, some patients may refuse in advance life-prolonging treatment, such as artificial nutrition and hydration after a severe stroke, in order to avoid becoming and remaining physically dependent on others for physical care.

What kind of complaint is made when an action or lack of it is said to be an offence against dignity? Arthur Frank is helpful here. He draws attention to the fact that there can be a spectrum of complaints in end of life care.[36] Some of these complaints may be more and some less serious than affronts to dignity. Frank suggests that 'dignity seems to be useful as a mid-level claim'. Hence, issues of dignity are likely to crop up in contexts in which someone's body and their feelings are in the control of others, or are very vulnerable to others, as is the case in end of life care. It does not require too much imagination, far less the need to go on a course, or to have a dignity measurement scale, to have an awareness as a nurse or physician of what observing the basic dignity of patients will require. In contrast 'special dignity', the dignity which stems from particular cultural or personal beliefs, does require some factual knowledge.

The concept of dignity can therefore be understood as follows. Respecting dignity requires certain basic forms of behaviour and treatment which we can all understand because we are all human—our patients are 'like us'. In addition there are certain cultural or personal beliefs which patients may have about how to treat them in a dignified way. We must ask about these. So understood dignity has a modest but definite role in the conceptual framework of end of life care.

From a philosophical perspective, dignity is a complex and controversial concept. Readers wishing to gain insight into this complexity and controversy may wish to read a review article in the *Journal of Medical Ethics*.[37]

9.3.ii Dignity, assisted suicide and euthanasia

We must finally return to the question of how this analysis of dignity bears on the issue of assisted suicide. Although dignity is an important concept in end of life care, there are limitations in its use. As Ruth Macklin points out: 'A pervasive problem with the concept of dignity is that it is used to defend and justify diametrically opposed actions or practices'.[38] She cites the example of voluntary euthanasia. In discussions of this, both proponents and opponents of voluntary euthanasia sometimes build their case round the concept of dignity. Thus, Pullman cites a Canadian Supreme Court ruling concerning PAS in which the justices on either side invoked human dignity.[39] The moral here may be the one drawn by Frank: that dignity is a mid-level claim, and cannot be used to settle high-level controversies.[40]

We are now in a position to answer various questions about dignity. Can it be defined? If by definition we mean a set of necessary and sufficient conditions then it cannot be defined. In particular it cannot be *restricted* to the ideas covered by self-determination or autonomy, although as rational, competent adults we have a right to be told the truth if we ask for it, and to give consent to treatment or refuse it. Again, it is an offence against dignity if we are not given a measure of privacy for basic bodily functions, or not given adequate pain relief.

Does dignity stretch beyond these basic contexts? Yes, the concept is to some extent culturally conditioned. It may be difficult from our own intuitions to know what a member of another culture might regard, say, as the dignified care of a body after death. This does not require a questionnaire, but a courteous discussion.[41]

Finally, how far can appeals to dignity settle fundamental controversies, such as whether or not assisted suicide or voluntary euthanasia should be legalized? The answer is not at all. Dignity cannot be used as a trump card in an argument; moreover, appeals to dignity can themselves be trumped by other considerations. For example, appealing to dignity to justify legalizing assisted suicide may be trumped by appeal to general social considerations (such as the possibility of abuse of any law governing PAS and euthanasia). But many people would disagree with that claim. Again, we shall leave it to the reader to decide.

9.4 A simple argument and a simple reply

In the end there are only two plausible arguments in favour of assisted suicide: the argument from unbearable suffering, and the argument from the desire for control.

First, there may be uncommon cases in which a person's suffering cannot be removed entirely despite the skills of specialists in palliative care. If such a person repeatedly requests euthanasia or assistance to commit suicide, then there is a strong case for saying that the request should be granted. This argument fits best the case of patients who have terminal illnesses or who face long-term illness with increasing symptoms and dependency. It turns on an empirical consideration—that the suffering cannot in fact be alleviated. New drugs or treatments might have the result that no suffering under medical supervision (as distinct from the battlefield, torture chamber, or burning lorry situations) could be called 'unbearable'. And of course what is or is not 'unbearable' is a subjective matter. For some people the situation of being dependent on others for care is perceived as 'unbearable'—this sort of deeply personal suffering is not amenable to drug treatment.

Second, there is the control argument. This argument is of much wider application and does not depend on an empirical premise. It might be said that someone who is, for example, paraplegic might reasonably judge that they have lost all control of their lives and simply want out of life. Others with progressive neurological deterioration, or facing a future of increasing cognitive decline, may judge that their current situation and future prospects are such that 'they would rather be dead'. Family members or the state may be willing to shoulder the burden of their care. But in the end if people with a serious degenerative disease, or recurrent psychiatric problems, whether terminal or not, just want their life to end is it morally wrong to grant their wish by either assisting them to kill themselves, or killing them oneself? This argument for PAS and euthanasia, based on enabling people to control the timing and method of their death, does not depend on a particular state of illness or prognosis; it rests instead simply on the desire that some people have to control the end of their lives. As Warnock and Macdonald put it, the issue is simply whether those who truly want death should 'have the right to die at someone else's hand, or with someone else's active cooperation.'[42]

Nevertheless, if assisting with suicide becomes a legal and socially legitimate activity, whether carried out by doctors or others, then the result is likely to be a lowering of the value of what has been regarded as sacred—life itself. But to erode social values in this way is to clear the ground for the obvious next step—taking the lives of those who have not requested it but are not in a position to resist it—the demented or the mentally handicapped, for example. This of course is the road that Nazi Germany went down. Hence, it might be said that we should not take the first step on that road. Another factor of moral relevance is the expectation that only a very small minority of people would actually take advantage of the availability of assistance in suicide or of euthanasia, whereas the effects (either benefit or harm) of legalization of these practices will be felt by the great majority as they eventually become dependent or require end of life care.

But it might be argued that the 'What kind of society do we want to live in?' arguments cut both ways. Do we want to live in a society in which people must continue to live in a physically dependent condition which they find deeply frustrating, with no prospect of recovery or other good outcome?

In conclusion, we also stress that the arguments about legalizing assisted suicide and euthanasia are not fundamentally about whether it might be 'right or wrong', morally justifiable or unjustifiable, to assist a particular individual to commit suicide or to kill that individual with euthanasia. Instead, they are about whether the proposed benefits (of alleviating suffering and making it easy for people to control the timing and manner of their death) actually outweigh the harms (of weakening society's prohibition of killing—especially by doctors—and putting pressure on those who are dependent or dying to end their lives so as to alleviate perceived or real burdens on others).

9.5 **Conclusions**

1. Arguments about withholding and withdrawing treatment or about sedation must be sharply distinguished from arguments about assisted suicide or voluntary euthanasia; the two sets of practices are not 'morally equivalent'.

2. 'The right to die' is a slogan which conceals many confusions.

3. The concept of human dignity is distinct from that of choice or self-determination.

4. Human dignity is an important ethical concept in end of life care, but it cannot be used as a trump card to settle important issues of public policy, such as the legalization of assisted suicide or voluntary euthanasia.

5. The strongest arguments in favour of legalizing assisted suicide and voluntary euthanasia are based on a claim of unbearable suffering or a desire to control one's life and one's death.

6. The strongest arguments against legalizing PAS and euthanasia are the likely weakening of the prohibition against killing (especially killing by doctors), and pressure (whether intended or not) on the sick to end their lives so as not to be a burden on others.

7. Most people have their own views on these matters and are not likely to be persuaded by further arguments. It is a matter for society to decide. But the involvement or otherwise of doctors in the acts of PAS and euthanasia ought to be for doctors themselves to decide.

References

1. Pereira J, Laurent P, Cantin B, Petremand D, Currat T (2008). The response of a Swiss university hospital's palliative care consult team to assisted suicide within the institution. *Palliative Medicine* **22**:659–67.

2. Saunders J (2006). What do physicians think about physician assisted suicide and voluntary euthanasia? *Clin Med* **8**:243–5.

3. Twisselmann B (2005). Time to legalise assisted dying? Summary of responses. *BMJ* **331**:843.

4. Gielen J, van den Branden S, Broeckaert B (2008). Attitudes of European physicians toward euthanasia and physician-assisted suicide: a review of the recent literature. *Journal of Palliative Care* **24**:173–84.

5. Montgomery J (2001). *Health care law*. Oxford University Press, Oxford, pp. 184–6.

6. General Medical Council (2002). *Withholding and withdrawing life-prolonging treatments*. GMC, London, para. 9.

7. British Medical Association (2007). *Withholding and withdrawing treatment life-prolonging medical treatment*, 3rd edn. Blackwell, Oxford, p. 3.

8. BMA, op. cit. (ref. 7), p. 3.

9. Warnock M, Macdonald E (2008). *Easeful death*. Oxford University Press, Oxford, p. 7.

10. Warnock, Macdonald, op. cit. (ref. 9), p. 20.

11. Warnock, Macdonald, op. cit. (ref. 9), p. xiv.

12. Warnock, Macdonald, op. cit. (ref. 9), p. 136.

13. Jenkins S (2008). Denial of the right to die is sheer religious primitivism. *Guardian*, 22 October 2008, p. 29.

14. Mcpherson CJ, Wilson KG, Lobchuk MM, Brajtman S (2007). Self-perceived burden to others: patient and family caregiver correlates. *Journal of Palliative Care* **23**:135–42.

15. Stone PC, Minton O (2008). Assisted dying: no change in the law is necessary. *British Journal of Hospital Medicine* **69**:434–5.

16. Available at http://news.bbc.co.uk1hi/health/4643196.stm (accessed on 31.12.08).

17. Grayling AC (2005). "Right to die". *BMJ* **330**:799.

18. Jenkins, op. cit. (ref. 13).

19. Warnock, Macdonald, op. cit. (ref. 9), p. ix.

20. Warnock, Macdonald, op. cit. (ref. 9), p. 7.

21. Warnock, Macdonald, op. cit. (ref. 9), p. 97.

22. Saunders J (2005). Assisted dying: considerations in the continuing debate. *Clin Med* **5**:543–7.

23. Saunders J (2006). Ethical decision-making in professional bodies. *Clin Med* **6**:13–15.

24. Savulescu J (2006). Conscientious objection in medicine. *BMJ* **332**:294.

25. Chervenak F, McCullough L, Smith VP (2006). Conscientious objection in medicine. *BMJ* **332**:425.

26. Smith M (2005). Patients and doctors: rights and responsibilities in the NHS (2). *Clin Med* **5**:501–2.

27. Commission for Healthcare Audit and Inspection (2007). *Caring for dignity*. CHAI, London, p. 57.

28. CHAI, op. cit. (ref. 27), p. 15.

29. Breitbart W, Chochinov HM, Passik SD (2004). Psychiatric symptoms in palliative medicine. In *Oxford textbook of palliative medicine*, 3rd edn. Oxford University Press, Oxford, pp. 757–8.

30. Chochinov HM (2002). Dignity-conserving care—a new model for palliative care. *J Am Med Assoc* **872**:2253–60.

31. Frank A (2004). Dignity, dialogue and care. *Journal of Palliative Care* **20**:207–11.

32. Pullman D (2004). Death, dignity and moral nonsense. *Journal of Palliative Care* **20**:174–8.

33. Tolstoy L [1886] (1960). *Death of Ivan Illich*. Penguin Classics, London.

34. Sophocles [*c*.492 BC] (1954). *Antigone*. Penguin Classics, London.

35. Pullman, op. cit. (ref. 32), p. 172.

36. Frank, op. cit. (ref. 31), p. 208.

37. Ashcroft R (2005). Making sense of dignity. *Journal of Medical Ethics* **31**:679–82.

38. Macklin R (2003). Dignity is a useless concept. *BMJ* **327**:1419–20.

39. Pullman, op. cit. (ref. 32), p. 171.

40. Frank, op. cit. (ref. 31), p. 208.

41. Chochinov H (2007). Dignity and the essence of medicine: the A, B, C, and D of dignity conserving care. *BMJ* **335**:184–7.

42. Warnock, Macdonald, op. cit. (ref. 9), p. 1.

Best interests: extended senses

In Part 1 we noted the uncontroversial obligation of health care professionals to act in the best interests of their patients. The 2008 consensus statement on the role of the doctor stipulates that 'The doctor's role must be defined by what is in the best interest of patients and of the population served.'[1] We consider that this statement would apply equally to other professionals engaged in end of life care, and that it rightly emphasizes the fundamental role of the concept of best interests in that care. Since the role and remit of health care professionals must be defined by 'the best interests of patients and the population served', we shall now consider further the scope and nature of 'best interests', and also whether the relatives should be included in 'the population served'. Both of these issues are controversial.

In Part 1 we assumed that the best interests of patients were promoted by means of the traditional aims of medicine: to prolong life, to alleviate suffering due to illness and to restore or maintain function. Our claim was that these remain the aims of end of life care, with the qualification that in pursuing the aims the priorities of care will alter, according to what is achievable and the patient's own priorities. So as the possibilities for prolonging life via treatment diminish, but the burdens and risks of that treatment remain significant, the aim of prolonging life very often rightly becomes subordinate to the aim of alleviating suffering. The British Medical Association noted that 'There needs to be a recognition that there comes a point in all lives where no more can reasonably or helpfully be done to benefit patients other than keeping them comfortable and free from pain.'[2] These changes in priorities frequently evolve gradually for both patients and professionals. Our belief in Part 1 of this book was that this approach to best interests expresses a consensus, as far as it goes.

In Part 2 we are considering the many views to the effect that our Part 1 interpretation of 'best interests' simply does not go far enough; that whereas prolonging life, alleviating suffering and restoring or maintaining function are certainly aspects of a patient's best interests, these interests are much wider and deeper, especially in end of life care. We have already discussed the view that a patient's best interests are furthered by advance care planning, including plans for the place of care and death. In this chapter we shall first examine the view that 'best interests' should be *extended* to include psychosocial and spiritual care. In short, that the aim of end of life care should be 'whole person' or 'holistic' care (Section 10.1). We include a brief discussion on the concept of 'meaning' and what makes life 'meaningful' (Section 10.2). Finally, we must examine the controversial view of specialist palliative care—included also in the 2008 *End of life care strategy*—that the unit of care is the patient and relatives, so the best interests of the relatives must also be considered. That issue will be the concern of Section 10.3.

10.1 'Best interests' extended to 'whole person' or 'holistic' care

It is sometimes said by those involved in end of life care that treatments/care, especially at the end of life, should take into account much more than physical and mental health issues. Treatments should be aimed not just at 'best interests' interpreted as achieving the three foundation aims in relation to illness, but at the patient's *overall* wellbeing. Such statements give rise to several important questions. For example, the World Health Organization (WHO) definition of palliative includes the identification, assessment and treatment of psychosocial and spiritual suffering.[3] How does 'whole person care' measure up as an enlarged interpretation of 'best interests'?

Wholeness, or overall wellbeing, is often said to be the ultimate goal of human life. Clearly, many things can go wrong as we all pursue this goal. Important among these mishaps is the occurrence of diseases and illnesses, both physical and mental. Alongside treatment of physical illness, the three foundation aims will encompass the treatment of mental states which are clearly pathological, such as anxiety states and major depression diagnosed at psychiatric assessment. But clearly there are many more impediments to the pursuit of wholeness than those which relate to physical and mental illness— such as emotional or spiritual distress, social isolation, or financial difficulties.

There is some professional expertise for dealing with spiritual and social problems. For example, the clergy may be able to soothe the troubled spirit, and social workers may be able to assist with making the case for financial assistance and improved housing. But there is a definite limitation on professional expertise in resolving or dealing with the natural human reactions of loss, sadness and anxiety associated with facing the end of life. This limitation is perhaps the main reason against making the pursuit of overall wellbeing an aim of health care. The achievement of wholeness by human beings may well be the supreme fulfilment of their best interests, but even the combined expertise of a team in health care is inadequate to achieve this aim!

Moreover, the aim of achieving wholeness in a patient would not be fulfilled by adding yet another set of experts. The reason for this is stated in Shakespeare's *Macbeth*:

Macbeth.	Canst thou not minister to a mind diseas'd,
	Pluck from the memory a rooted sorrow,
	Raze out the written troubles of the brain,
	And with some sweet oblivious antidote
	Cleanse the stuff'd bosom of that perilous stuff
	Which weighs upon the heart?
Doctor.	Therein the patient
	Must minister to himself.[4]

In other words, Shakespeare is saying that we cannot make any helpful impact on the psychological, social or spiritual condition of another, unless the subject is actively involved. The subjects cannot be passive in this process—if they are the attempt is bound to be ineffective. By contrast, physical illness can be influenced by external factors such as drugs or technological interventions without much active participation by the patient, and health care professionals reasonably bear responsibility for provision of such treatment. Whereas it is clear that a patient's interests will ultimately extend beyond the relief of illness-related suffering to the achievement of wholeness or overall wellbeing, health care must be modest in what it claims it can do to improve the social, psychological and spiritual aspects of a patient's interests. The professional team can influence those interests only in partnership with the patient. The patient (unless mentally ill) has by far the most control over his or her own psychological wellbeing.

It might be said that even if professionals have little control over the emotional state of a patient, they should at least try to understand that state. Sometimes this kind of understanding is called 'empathy'. Experts working in the field of end of life care and bereavement have described empathy as 'being able to sense accurately and appreciate another person's reality and to convey that understanding sensitively.'[5] But there is a problem with saying that there is a professional duty to achieve empathy or that staff can be trained to empathize. No doubt some staff can sometimes achieve this sort of understanding with some patients, but the belief that we can routinely empathize, or indeed be trained to empathize, is a dangerous illusion. Those attempting to provide training/education in empathy advise techniques such as repetition and paraphrasing of the patient's words, and naming the patient's feelings, to 'indicate that we are listening and trying to understand.'[6] Although these techniques are designed to impress upon the patient that we are trying to understand, they in no way actually enable us to 'sense accurately and appreciate another person's reality'.

It is hard enough to understand someone with whom one has lived for twenty years; the possibility of truly understanding a patient is therefore remote. But just as it is possible to love completely without complete understanding, so it is possible to give humane treatment without complete emotional understanding.

The important point is that we must respect the patient as an individual unique among others. This means listening to the patient's own preferences, priorities, and overall perspective. Professionals then take these into account when selecting treatment options, so as to present the patient with those options which are clinically the most appropriate to achieve the patient's goals and values as these relate to the three aims of health care. The selection of treatment options, and the way that they are presented to the patient, both require the exercise of *clinical judgement*. It follows that the exercise of this clinical judgement is a moral imperative; such judgement should qualify any intervention in end of life care, and it must also underlie the concept of whole person care.

Paradoxically, it is precisely the fact that whole person care implies respect for the patient's own personal preferences and priorities, goals and values that imposes limits on the scope of professional activity directed towards such care. We must not attempt to inflict unwanted attention or solutions to emotional or social problems on patients, any more than we would inflict unwanted physical treatment without patients' adequately informed consent. Recognition of this limitation is an integral part of the concept of whole person care, because included in this concept is the control individuals always have over their own psychological, social, and spiritual integrity. Thus professionals must accept that no assessment or intervention can be given which the informed patient with capacity does not want. Where a patient lacks capacity, professionals should refrain from intervening in psychosocial or spiritual issues unless there is good reason to believe that the patient would have wanted the intervention. The requirement for consent in relation to physical interventions is well recognized, but it is sometimes forgotten or regarded with less respect in terms of psychosocial and spiritual care. In all forms of care it is an ethical necessity to respect a patient's wishes in relation to whether or not an assessment or intervention is acceptable; such respect is integral to the concept of whole person care.

Recognition of the limits to psychosocial and spiritual care must also be underlined because it acts as a safeguard against the setting of unrealistic goals for the patient and the team. If those limits are not recognized, there is a risk that patients, their relatives, and the professional team may expect that end of life care can alleviate, and ought to alleviate, all suffering which has its basis in psychological, social and spiritual issues. There is currently a lack of recognition of the limits to professional ability to determine or change a patient's psychosocial or spiritual condition. This is not a question of lack of expertise in using interventions (such as lack of skill in using drugs or in practical procedures) but is instead a question of lack of effective interventions in the first place! There is also perhaps inadequate discussion of whether it is really appropriate to try to alter a patient's psychosocial condition when the latter is a normal, and probably appropriate, response to circumstances. As Iona Heath comments in her book *Matters of life and death*: 'By implying that dying can be detached from suffering, medicine makes a false promise and devalues, as somehow obsolete and unnecessary, the age-old human endeavour of facing pain and suffering with fortitude and stoicism. This seems a very serious error'.[7] These matters are of such ethical importance and cause such controversy that we shall discuss them further now.

The *End of life care strategy* optimistically stipulates that all acute hospitals must have 'mechanisms to ensure that relevant healthcare professionals have the necessary competences . . . to elicit priorities and preferences and to meet physical, psychological, social and spiritual end of life care needs.'[8] The belief (by all concerned) that professionals ought to be able to meet all psychological, social and spiritual end of life care needs, presumably leading to a state of overall wellbeing for the patient, is completely unrealistic. There are surely no 'competences' which could achieve the goal of overall psychological, social and spiritual wellbeing for or with patients. Indeed, attempts to achieve this goal are likely to lead not only to disappointment, frustration and guilt, but also sometimes to inappropriate 'assessment' and 'treatment' of normal human reactions to the end of life situation.

This last concern is of considerable ethical importance in end of life care because of the concurrence of two factors, namely the current stress placed on psychosocial and spiritual assessment and intervention by professionals, and the tendency to treat any mental state considered as 'depression' with either medication or counselling or even both. Individuals facing the end of their lives confront many psychological and social anxieties, and also confront major losses such as independence, the leaving of loved ones and life itself. Experiencing such losses will give rise to the normal human responses of sadness in most people. There is a concern that this normal sadness, which is not a mental disorder or mental illness, may not be differentiated from the mental disorder of depression. Instead, it may be assessed and treated as if it were depression with some adverse consequences. Similarly, normal anxieties may not be differentiated from pathological anxiety states.

Professor Allan Horwitz, a social scientist, and Professor Jerome Wakefield, a social worker, have recently pointed out that it is important to distinguish between the human responses of anxiety and sadness, which are normal and possibly adaptive in certain external circumstances, and pathological anxiety states and depression which are 'maladaptive' responses and are 'disordered'.[9] They argue that normal sadness brought on by external circumstances is increasingly being diagnosed as 'depression' because the current diagnostic criteria for the latter mental illness are based on the identification of symptoms such as depressed mood, loss of appetite and fatigue lasting for at least two weeks.[10] But these symptoms are also associated with intense normal sadness. These authors noted that the 'separation of normal sadness and depressive disorder is a sensible and legitimate, indeed a crucial one . . . it has both clinical and scientific importance.' They went on to express concern that the recent loss of this distinction is resulting in 'classifying many instances of normal sadness as mental disorders.'[11] In normal sadness, the response is due to the context, is of roughly proportionate intensity to the provoking loss, and it either ends when the loss situation ends or it gradually ceases as coping mechanisms adjust.[12] They pointed out that the appropriate response to normal sadness 'was to offer support, to help the individual cope and move on despite the loss, and to avoid confusing the person's sadness with illness.' By contrast, the depressive conditions of mental illness are disproportionate to external events and circumstances, tend to be long-lasting and recurrent, are due to some internal dysfunction and require professional attention.[13]

In end of life care, loss of the distinction between normal sadness (not a mental disorder) and depression (a mental disorder) gives rise to ethical issues in both assessment of psychosocial state and in subsequent intervention or treatment.

Taking assessment first, professionals in end of life care are told to focus on psychological wellbeing and they are advised to make routine attempts to elicit signs of depression.[14] Guidance on psychosocial aspects of palliative care recommends the routine use of screening questions to detect depression (followed by routine use of anti-depressants and cognitive behavioural therapy if screening is positive).[15] Two simple questions are advocated as an initial 'pre-screening' test. Patients are asked whether in the last month (or perhaps 2 weeks) they have been bothered by having 'little interest or pleasure in doing things' and by 'feeling down, depressed or hopeless.'[16] Ideally, if the patient answers 'yes' to either or both of these questions a proper psychiatric assessment should follow to determine whether the patient is depressed and to offer appropriate treatment. Given the standard psychiatric symptom criteria (such as the American Psychiatric Association's *Diagnostic and statistical manual of mental disorders*, 4th edition (DSM-IV)), which apply regardless of the context of the patient's circumstances, a diagnosis of depression is quite likely to follow such assessment. In reality, psychiatric assessments are less likely to occur in end of life care because of the resource requirements in terms of patients' energy and psychiatrists' time. Instead, professionals may rely only on the two questions plus perhaps using a brief questionnaire[17] based on the DSM-IV criteria, possibly resulting in an even higher rate of diagnosis of depression.

Such 'screening processes' applied to cancer patients lead to high rates of diagnosis of depression; when the most 'stringent' psychiatric criteria are applied, 5–15% of patients will meet criteria for major depression and a further 10–15% present with less severe symptoms which are said to 'require treatment', according to guidance from palliative care.[18] So apparently 20–30% have 'depression' requiring treatment! This result is perhaps not surprising as the same guidance notes that minor depression requires only two to four symptoms to qualify for diagnosis.

But as Horwitz and Wakefield pointed out, many of the symptoms which occur in non-disordered normal sadness also occur in depression. So using symptom-based diagnosis for depression without attention to the context of the patient's symptoms results in 'the pathologization of normal sadness' because many patients who are in fact understandably sad, will instead be diagnosed as being depressed.[19] This is particularly likely to occur when 'pre-screening' questions or brief questionnaires are used in the context of end of life care.[20] Furthermore there is no 'gold standard', such as a biological test, which could differentiate between people who are normally sad (and not disordered) and those who are depressed—so in end of life care there is no way to ensure that normal people are not wrongly diagnosed as disordered, i.e. suffering from depression.[21]

An alternative psychiatric diagnosis of 'adjustment disorder' is sometimes used to describe clinically significant behavioural or emotional symptoms occurring as a result of some trigger or stressor, for example severe chronic and terminal illness. Adjustment disorder is said to be a maladaptive response which is 'highly prevalent' according to authors advising on psychosocial palliative care. They criticize oncologists for failing to diagnose adjustment disorder, but they also admit that it is a rather 'nebulous disorder', that it is 'difficult to define what constitutes maladaptive behaviour especially under circumstances of monumental stress' and that there is no quick and easy method for detecting it. Despite these major uncertainties they claim that 'comorbidity of psychiatric diagnosis and cancer diagnosis should be viewed as the rule rather than the exception',[22] thus implying (somewhat implausibly) that most patients with cancer have a psychiatric illness! Other authors have warned that 'If applied too loosely, the diagnosis of adjustment disorder can pathologize the experience of some patients by applying a psychiatric label on what may be a normal experience of grief.'[23]

The conclusion for end of life care is obvious—assessment of psychosocial wellbeing, particularly by 'screening' using abbreviated assessments, is likely to result in diagnosis of depression or adjustment disorder in many people who are normal and not disordered.

But there is also a more pervasive and serious moral consequence for us all, as was noted by Horwitz and Wakefield: when mood symptoms are assessed without attention to their context, 'all normal sadness responses potentially can be seen as a sign of pathology; the very possibility of normal sadness is lost.'[24] (We shall mention this observation again with reference to bereavement.)

Turning now to interventions/treatment, there is clearly a danger that the ideal of whole person care combined with assessments of psychosocial state could lead professionals to 'treat' normal sorrows as if they were a mental illness. Indeed, treatment of feelings of sadness seems to be recommended by authors advising on palliative care.[25] These authors note that depressive symptoms are estimated to be present in a quarter of cancer patients, and they recommend drug treatment. But this policy may lead to 'treatment' which, although appropriate for the mental disorder of depression, is not necessarily appropriate for normal sadness. Similar concerns surround the distinction between normal anxiety and adjustment disorder.

It might be objected that treating normal sadness as depression in the end of life situation may not be a morally bad outcome, as the 'treatment' might reduce the patient's distress. But there are three counter-arguments to this objection. The first is that anti-depressants have side-effects and it has been noted that the evidence of benefit from anti-depressants in minor depression is not convincing.[26,27] The second is that patients wrongly identified as depressed may feel alarmed, stigmatized, and not motivated to comply with the treatment, especially if they do not regard themselves as suffering from a disorder. The third is the major moral consequence of regarding normal sadness as something which should be 'treated' so as to attempt to abolish it via health care interventions, while health care professionals come to believe that they have a duty to try to ensure the patient's overall psychological, social and spiritual wellbeing.[28] This consequence is particularly likely if assessment and treatment recommended in the palliative care literature is widely implemented in end of life care.

Whole person care does imply responsibility for the diagnosis and treatment of true physical and mental illness states, yet it surely does not entail treating normal human reactions to the end of life situation as though they were mental illnesses!

Fortunately there are two potential solutions which might avoid this individual and social adverse outcome. The first pertains to the process of consent, and the second to certain aspects of the professional's role.

We have already noted the importance of obtaining the patient's consent prior to assessment and intervention regarding psychosocial or spiritual states. If having given such consent the patient is found to have symptoms of sadness and low mood, the patient should be informed about the extreme difficulty of differentiating between normal sadness and depression, and about the lack of convincing evidence for the use of anti-depressants in minor depression and depression in severe physical illness.[29,30] If the professional considers that anti-depressants should be offered as they hold a reasonable prospect of net benefit despite the uncertainties, then the patient is sufficiently informed about the situation to make a decision whether to accept such medication or not. The same requirements for information would apply to the use of counselling techniques/treatments, as evidence for these is limited.[31]

The second solution pertains to our human relationship with the patient. Whole person care implies a willingness to assist the patient to overcome psychological, social, and spiritual barriers to wellbeing, by using our relationship with them as fellow members of a community. In this last task we are acting not so much in our professional roles but more as a caring companion who has had the benefit of listening to the experiences and feelings of many previous patients in similar situations. Alongside our professional role, it can be argued that we have this role as a concerned fellow human being who will support the patient by continuing to listen to concerns, not flinching from ongoing distress, and sometimes by assisting the patient to identify what can still be hoped for in their personal goals.

Dr Iona Heath, in a chapter on 'What the doctor needs', writes eloquently about the relationship between doctor and dying patient.[32] What she is describing is a relationship of human companionship, not a professional expertise that could be acquired through training. She mentions the importance of being willing to look directly at the patient, not avoiding eye contact. She asks 'How is it—precisely—that some doctors and nurses are able to convey their presence and lack of flinching, while others turn away? Is it through words or touch or silence or all of these, or none, or something else—is it possible to say?'

With regard to what is said, she acknowledges that one person cannot have a direct experience of another's pain, so each must depend on words and on the listener's imagination. She observes that 'The nature of the relationship between speaker and listener determines how much can be communicated . . . . We can pay healing attention to fear only if we can locate it and, as doctors, we can discover it only by inviting words, by listening and by carefully and deliberately imagining.' Her summary of how we should use our eyes, words, touch and patience to promote healing in the care of the dying is realistic, accurate and moving for clinicians—we recognize in it what has been 'good' about the good care we may have achieved with some of our dying patients. It is all to do with our humanity.

But there is a fine line between providing companionable support and intruding destructively. As Heath also notes in a chapter entitled 'How is it possible to die?', for many patients it is necessary to review their own story, and for some, making sense of it and perhaps finding some personal meaning will help them to accept death. Professionals must be careful not to intrude destructively, or assume understanding where there is none.[33] We can watch for ways to be useful in the patient's own exploration, and give tactful support where it is wanted.

It is as a result of both the professional and the companionship role that patients tend to feel that their worth as individuals has been affirmed. Any person in the health care team treating them competently and compassionately, with respect for their preferences and values, can aid such affirmation. Patients also feel that their worth is affirmed when society in some way provides resources for their care at the end of life, even though recovery is not possible and they are likely to become or remain dependent on others for care. In these ways end of life care can affirm the value of each patient, promoting and not inhibiting overall wellbeing, even when independence is lost.

A good case can be made for giving a cautious acceptance to the concept of whole person or holistic care as an extension of the concept of best interests. It can encapsulate the basic aims of end of life care—such as the relief of suffering—and also involve the offer of help for emotional, spiritual, or relationship problems. It should be acknowledged, however, that the support given in addressing psychosocial and spiritual problems is not mainly based on professional expertise, but on the attention and perhaps even wisdom of a compassionate and experienced human being. It might in fact be less misleading (and so preferable) to speak of the 'humane' professional and humane care, rather than the 'holistic' professional and holistic care. But the term 'holistic' is endemic in end of life care literature.

The essential safeguard is to remember the ethical rule that we ought to respect the values of other unique individuals who may or may not want professional involvement in the psychological, social and spiritual aspects of their lives which are necessarily deeply personal and central to their integrity. Patients' values, or their interests as they perceive them, may not correspond to their emotional or spiritual interests as seen by the team. Professional help can only be offered; if it is to be of benefit it must be in partnership with the patient. Patients' adequately informed consent should be sought before involvement by professionals—this entails information about what can and cannot be achieved in psychosocial and spiritual care, and about the many uncertainties. The context of end of life care does not justify imposing on patients unwanted professional assessment, involvement or intervention.

There have been suggestions (for example, in the WHO definition of palliative care) that the aim of end of life care should be improvement of the patient's and family's quality of life; we have argued against replacing 'best interests' with 'quality of life' in our previous work.[34]

This takes us to the question of what should be the aim(s) or goal(s) of end of life care? In answering this question we shall suggest the direction in which we believe end of life care philosophy and practice should develop—back to the aims of all health care! We suggest that the 'best interests' goals in end of life care should be: the alleviation of symptoms due to illness; the maximization of functioning; and the prolongation of life. The WHO came to similar conclusions in 2004 in an evidence-based report on palliative care. They concluded that simple measures, including pain and symptom relief, sensitive communication of clear information, and well coordinated care, are effective in relieving symptoms and suffering, and 'can help people live meaningfully until the end of life'.[35]

10.2 Meaning and dignity at the end of life

Most people at some time ask themselves questions such as the following: What does my life add up to? Have I ever done anything really worthwhile? In the last phase of life people might ask themselves such questions with more urgency. These questions must be distinguished from equally natural questions about the mode or processes of dying. Questions of the latter sort are scientific questions which, however important, we shall not address here. Questions of the former sort concern what makes life and death of significance to people and gives meaning to life and death.

The term 'spiritual' is now preferred to the term 'religious' regarding these ultimate questions. The reason for this is that while the origins of palliative care were in religious orders, contemporary professionals wish to appeal to a much wider constituency. They therefore use the word 'spiritual' since it covers the wider issues. A definition by Carl Attwood, a clergyman involved in palliative care, illustrates this: 'a helpful definition broadens spirituality to cover that non-material part of a person's life which is concerned with their understanding of meaning and truth both about themselves and of their place in the world.'[36] Now, questions of this spiritual nature, concerning the meaningful life, may receive answers of two different sorts. The first we can deal with reasonably easily, but the second is much harder.

The first set of questions arises when spirituality takes a religious form. Many people still have religious beliefs. Even if the beliefs have lain dormant for many years they may well re-awaken in the last phase of life. When such patients desire help, the responsibility for offering comfort, explanation, reassurance, and sometimes help to clarify or reinforce their beliefs, really rests with the clergy because of their vocation, knowledge and skill. For those who sincerely hold a religious belief, what gives their life meaning is something which comes from outside them. What is important to stress here is that for such patients their lives are *given* meaning; they can see their lives as part of a larger framework. As Carl Attwood notes (see above) 'for some [spirituality] is essentially about the spirit that can be acted upon by, and reflect, the Divine.' The often asked question 'Why me?' can then be answered by references to God's overall plans and purposes for human life. Even though the task of the clergy may sometimes be difficult, there is no theoretical problem about the aim. Clergy and religious advisers are available in hospitals, hospices and the community, so professionals providing end of life care need not be mainly involved here.

We must note, however, that many people do not have such religious beliefs. For them their lives are not given meaning from the outside. Spiritual meaning must therefore be found in the way their lives are lived and ended. What are the factors which make a life seem meaningful? This raises the second and more complex set of issues. The issues are partly conceptual: certain factors make a life *count* as meaningful. Someone whose main activities are gambling and spending the proceeds on himself might have an exciting or enjoyable life, but it hardly counts as a meaningful life. The factors are partly empirical or experiential: the adoption of certain purposes *causes* people to feel that their lives are meaningful. For example, someone who trains for and obtains a job may feel that his life is meaningful, and experiences such as falling in love or sharing an interest with a friend can also cause us to feel that our lives are meaningful. The factors are partly *moral*: for we morally approve of the meaningful life and withhold the term 'meaningful' from lives which lack certain purposes or qualities. An embezzler might be very skilful, but we would not call his life meaningful. Whatever contributes to the meaningful life must be morally acceptable.

Granted the acceptability of this three-aspect analysis we are left with the question of what can be said to patients in the final phase of their lives if they seek reassurance about these anxieties when facing death. But not all patients want such reassurance; if they do, they may not wish to receive it from doctors, nurses or therapists. It would be quite wrong to imply to patients, whatever the motivation, that relief of physical symptoms is in any way tied to discussion of these possible end of life anxieties. But for those patients who do wish such discussion there is some general advice from Dame Cicely Saunders: patients at the ends of their lives should live until they die. Our questions, then, are: What are the purposes, the activities, the conversations which would count as a meaningful end to a life, which would cause or enable someone to feel that their life has ended in a meaningful or worthwhile way, which would be morally good, and which would enable them to 'live until they die'?

It is obvious, but perhaps should be stated, that to be meaningful is not the same as to be profound or socially important. Ordinary activities and relationships are what are likely to constitute a meaningful end to a life, especially when the person is already very sick. Hence, our suggestions may be obvious or banal, but it is worth stressing that professionals should not try to be over-ambitious. Carl Attwood's paper gives helpful and realistic guidance. There is a tendency to assume that bad relationships must be put right at the end of life, but this may not be possible for a variety of reasons, and perhaps it is a mistake to encourage attempts that may fail, especially if the attempt is exhausting. The idea of a good death or a meaningful end may sometimes be more in the minds of professionals than patients! Nevertheless, a few points can be made.

First of all, visits from friends and relatives are important for most patients. Iona Heath describes the value of retelling and reliving important events with family. She also mentions the importance for the patient of being able to review the life, make an account, and to salve bad memories and allow for expressions of remorse and forgiveness.[37] Clergymen may have an important role here, if the patient wishes, as Carl Attwood notes. Some patients want a final trip home or to a place of emotional significance.

For some patients the consciousness that life is coming to an end can spark off creative ability which has lain dormant for a lifetime. It is through the arts that some patients can express what they find difficult to say, and some specialist palliative care units employ art or music therapists, or have a writer or artist in residence, to aid such expression. Other patients may wish to contribute to the general good by taking part in research. Professionals may be protective of their patients and so may resist outside attempts to encourage frail patients to participate in clinical trials. Nevertheless, some patients may wish to enter trials as a way of contributing to a morally good project.

If we turn now to the connected idea of dignity at the end of life we find that the ability to exercise some marginal control over one's life, to exercise some choice, is often depicted as important. As we have seen in Chapter 8 the truth in this has been trivialized by those who suggest that dying in the place of your choice is the key factor in dignity at the end of life, and who therefore wish to make it the primary 'performance measure'. Surely the *place* of death is not likely to be the only or the most important factor contributing to a dignified death. In any case, we are emphatically not going down the path of many, perhaps the vast majority of those concerned with end of life ethics, who make choice an essential factor for human dignity (see Section 9.3.i). Even when no choices are possible, life can be given significance by an acceptance of the inevitable. Human dignity in end of life care is often shown through courage, humour, and concern for others. The poet Andrew Marvell, in describing the execution of Charles I, provides a portrait of dignity where no choice was available:

> He nothing common did, or mean,
> Upon that memorable scene;
> But bowed his comely head
> Down, as upon a bed.[38]

We conclude that there are many ways, other than by granting their choices, in which patients can be helped to feel that their lives are meaningful, and many ways in which dignity can be shown and respected.

10.3 **Best interests and relatives**

Professional codes of conduct for doctors and nurses do not include statements about any obligations to relatives, only obligations to patients. We noted at the beginning of this chapter that the recent consensus statement on the role of the doctor mentions only obligations to patients—the only possibility for inclusion of relatives would be a tenuous and controversial interpretation of 'the population served'. The International Labour Organization definitions of the roles of doctors and nurses do not include obligations or activities with relatives of patients.[39]

Moreover, it is clear in professional codes of conduct that obligations of confidentiality towards patients override requests from relatives for information—so long as the patient has capacity, the information should not be disclosed without the patient's consent. Similarly, treatment selection must be based on patients' interests, not those of relatives, and when adults with capacity consent to or refuse a treatment relatives cannot countermand or subvert that decision. These codes are widely accepted by health care professionals in the Western world, and are implicitly accepted by the communities which fund and use health services. Professional codes are coherent with law, which in practice supports them. The law does not state that there is a duty of care to the relatives. Many laws (including UK law) are explicit that decisions for patients who lack capacity must be based only on the patient's best interests (and therefore not on the interests of relatives).

Nevertheless, despite the concurrence of ethical codes and law, the belief in obligations to relatives is rarely questioned in specialist palliative care. This is shown by statements such as the following, contained in a systematic review of the level of need for palliative care: 'Clearly, palliative care services must address the psychological as well physical symptoms associated with the disease process, not only in the patient, but also in the family units supporting the patient.'[40] The WHO definition of palliative care clearly implies that the aim of improving the quality of life of the family is as important as the same aim for patients.

Moreover, the recent *End of life care strategy* strongly recommends professional involvement with 'carers' and 'family members' of patients, both those providing care for the patient and those who are not. The strategy stipulates that 'carers' should be offered a professional assessment of their needs and a formal 'carer's care plan' which may be separate from the care plan for the patient. The strategy also stipulates that family members and carers should be given information about the illness, including its likely course, but it does not even acknowledge the issue of confidentiality in such disclosure. It alludes to conflicts of interest between patient and family by stating simply, 'Family members may have needs for psychological and social support that are separate from those of the carer or the person who is being cared for. It should also be recognised that the carer's needs and wishes may conflict with those of the dying person and perhaps the rest of the family and will need to be managed carefully.'[41] In its recommendations, including the stipulation that carers should be offered a 'care plan' for themselves, the strategy is effectively stating that there is a *duty of care to the family*. Such a duty of care establishes a 'therapeutic' relationship between professional and family, with associated obligations.

Why do influential groups take this approach for end of life care, in the face of the traditional focus on the patient in all other aspects of health care? The (alleged) health benefits of including the family in the unit of care are explained in texts on palliative care. The *Oxford textbook of palliative medicine* (OTPM) states that 'while the patient experiences greater physical symptoms, family caregivers often experience a greater degree of suffering as they observe the patient'.[42] The OTPM, in its chapter on bereavement, notes in relation to the professional role that 'Family-centred care is integral to this supportive process as the family's understanding of the illness and its treatment influences their later adjustment'.[43] Thus the first benefit is the reduction in suffering of family caregivers during the patient's life, and the second is the promotion of the interests of the family in bereavement. Since there are links between the relatives' experience of the patient's terminal illness and their subsequent bereavement, we are discussing both of these alleged benefits in this section. In 10.4.ii we shall comment on the evidence for the claims of reduction in relatives' suffering in bereavement.

But before considering such evidence, we shall question whether a plausible case can be made for professional obligations to relatives, and if so, how far ought those obligations to extend?

10.3.i The nature and extent of obligations to relatives

The idea that the wellbeing of relatives is part of the remit of end of life care is now entrenched, and so it is not surprising that it is the focus of the entire fifth chapter of the *End of life care strategy*. It is also very unlikely that other new guidance on end of life care without any such mention would be accepted. Granted this situation, the statement about any obligations to relatives must be explicit about the nature of such obligations and their limits.

The aims of end of life care—its distinctive contributions to human welfare—are to relieve the suffering of patients, to prolong their lives if that is possible and their wish, and to provide for their nursing care needs. But because of their unique position and relationship with a given patient, professionals are likely also to be in contact with the family. It is therefore entirely appropriate and fitting, and indeed an obligation, that they should offer words of comfort to the family. They should be 'friendly professionals'. Being a 'friendly professional' does not require 'expertise', but it does require moral and emotional maturity, and the expression of this professional concern and friendship comprises the first type of general obligation to relatives.[44]

Second, relatives should be given information and explanation about the illness within the constraints of confidentiality to patients. Moreover they should be given realistic reassurance, encouragement and advice when they are participating in the patient's care. But such support should be given with due regard to the time required and the opportunity cost to patients.

Third, when patients lack capacity and treatment decisions are required, relatives should be asked about the patient's previously stated wishes, feelings, beliefs and values, what they think the patient would have wanted, and their opinion about the patient's best interests. If possible, their agreement should be reached with the treatment plan. But the patient's interests should not be significantly compromised in order to reach such agreement (see Section 2.5).

Fourth, there are obligations to relatives to warn them about possible harms to themselves. Relatives caring for patients at home often run the risk of physical injury, especially through trying to lift the patient using risky techniques or without the appropriate lifting aids. In order to protect relatives from physical injury and exhaustion, there is an obligation to provide necessary equipment and practical nursing care input so long as the agreed care plan is for the patient to remain at home. Having said this, the issue of the *extent* of the obligation to avoid harm to relatives who are caring for a patient at home remains ethically problematic.

We discussed in Chapter 8 the considerable ethical problems of the harms which family carers may sustain when the patient's preference for being at home is met. Where that care continues for months or even years (for example when the patient has dementia) there is a risk of real physical and emotional exhaustion for family carers, whose health and integrity of emotional wellbeing may be threatened by the burdens of care even when outside assistance is provided.

Professionals, patients and families are now faced with ethical problems and apparently with no solutions; there is current enthusiasm (plus some political pressure) to meet patients' preferences to be at home, no matter what their care needs or the burdens on others, while at the same time the new strategy on end of life care has effectively confirmed a professional duty of care to the family. It will not be possible always (or even often) to negotiate away the conflict of interest between patients and families. Yet no guidance is given on how this conflict should be resolved. Professionals therefore face the possibility of being seen to fail in a duty of care to either patient or family where this situation occurs. With regard to the single issue of location of care and (particularly) death, the interests of family carers appear to have been subordinated to those of the patient. It is ethically inconsistent to create a duty of care to the family and then to apparently negate that duty by considering that on this single issue the patient's wishes must necessarily override the interests of caring family members.

There are two possible explanations for the apparent inconsistency. The first is that the authors of the *End of life care strategy* may not in fact believe that there is a duty of care to the family members and/or family carers of the patient. Such a position would be consistent with the law and professional codes of conduct, and with the principle that decisions for patients lacking capacity must be based only on the patient's best interests. But if this is the case it would have been far preferable not to have effectively stipulated a duty of care to the family and thus implied a therapeutic relationship between professionals and the family, with its attendant obligations. The second possible explanation is that there is some sort of duty to protect carers from harm and to support them in their caring role, but the achievement of the patient's preference for location of care and death (when that preference is home) is deemed to be of such great importance that it should override consideration of adverse effects on family carers.

We conclude that there is an obligation to provide physical assistance to family members in their care of the patient at home, and to try to prevent injury to them. But the issue of whether the interests of family carers should be considered in the decision regarding place of care for the patient remains controversial and unresolved. Two factors are relevant: first, location of care and death is not a patient-treatment decision (with associated professional obligations); second, in ordinary morality we do not normally consider that the interests of one person should necessarily override the interests of others. So why should the interests of a person approaching the end of life necessarily override those of their family carers when location of care is the issue at stake? There surely cannot be a new professional obligation to ensure that patients are cared for and die in the place of their choice—it is implausible because it is unachievable. By contrast, a plausible case can be made for considering the welfare of family carers in decisions about location of care and death for the patient, especially as consideration must be given to what the health service can reasonably provide in terms of professional care at home. We leave readers to consider the arguments for themselves.

From the above discussion we suggest that there are some obligations to relatives, but they are quite different from obligations which arise from the special therapeutic relationship between professional and patient.

None the less we acknowledge that those approaching the issue from a specialist palliative care point of view tend to see the relatives as of *therapeutic* concern, which implies a therapeutic relationship and associated obligations (it has been recommended that relatives be seen as 'secondary patients'[45]). They then face inevitable conflicts with obligations to patients. The *End of life care strategy* position is ethically similar. This position remains inconsistent with professional codes and law; it is ethically problematic for end of life care to be out of step with the rest of health care in this respect. In addition, it becomes even more difficult to justify if, as we shall see, the evidence for the effectiveness of current policy in promoting welfare in bereavement is weak.

10.3.ii Bereavement care: benefit or harm?

Following a review of available evidence, the WHO in 2004 stated that there is relatively little evidence for the predictive power of assessments to determine the need for support and counselling after bereavement, or for the benefit of individual bereavement support. The WHO acknowledged that these interventions are difficult to evaluate.[46] NICE in its evidence-based guidance on palliative care for adults with cancer (2004) similarly acknowledged that risk assessment tools cannot be relied upon as a predictor of bereavement outcome, and that 'evidence for one-to-one therapeutic interventions is currently unclear'.

Yet it still recommended that services be provided to focus on the needs of families in bereavement.[47] The 2008 *End of life care strategy* recommends early assessment of the needs of individual family members for bereavement support, although it acknowledges that there is only 'some evidence to suggest' that this is effective preventative health care.[48] It goes on to recommend that bereavement care and support should be offered to and be available for *all* carers, family members and close friends of the patient.[49] The controversial questions for us now are whether bereavement requires assessment, and whether bereavement support should be more generally available for all those close to the patient in end of life care.

It has been estimated that about 10% of bereaved people have enduring symptoms which constitute a depressive disorder, known as 'complicated grief', for which professional intervention is appropriate.[50] But this does not mean that there is any justification for trying to assess the risk of complicated grief in *every* bereaved relative, and setting up services which will follow up *every* bereaved relative. Yet strangely, this is what the *End of life care strategy* recommends. The 2002 WHO definition of palliative care similarly advocates the assessment and treatment of psychosocial suffering in the patient's family plus bereavement counselling if necessary.[51]

Given the uncertainties surrounding the ability to identify family members at risk of abnormal or abnormally severe bereavement reactions, and very limited evidence of benefit from one-to-one bereavement support, it seems impossible to justify subjecting families to formal assessments of their risk for morbid bereavement outcome, or the resources expended in such assessments, or the provision of one-to-one bereavement support (with the associated resource consequences) outside of research projects. The exception would be treatment for the small minority of people who are identified as suffering from complicated grief after bereavement, since evidence supports such intervention.[52]

Indeed, there is a plausible case for saying that both the process of risk assessment for pathological bereavement, and routine provision of bereavement counselling, may actually do harm.

Authors with considerable experience in bereavement work have noted that intrusive procedures to assess the risk of morbid bereavement can do harm, and have warned against their use.[53] We have already noted the lack of evidence for their effectiveness.

It is also acknowledged that bereavement counselling itself can do harm. A *BMJ* editorial in 2007 noted that people going through normal or uncomplicated grief after a death usually do not benefit from anything other than general support, and cited evidence indicating that specific interventions may be contraindicated.[54] Several kinds of harm might result from such inappropriate bereavement counselling.

First, assertions (such as the WHO definition of palliative care) that psychosocial suffering due to feelings of grief, misery, anger, and loneliness must be relieved by identification, assessment and treatment of these states of mind may in themselves be damaging. These states are normal human reactions to the loss of a major bereavement—they are not sickness or disease. David Kissane, writing in the OTPM, comments that 'For the majority, although bereavement is painful, their personal resilience will ensure their normal adaptation. There can, therefore, be no justification for routine intervention as grief is not a disease.'[55] Earlier in this chapter we referred to the morally significant social consequences of treating normal sadness responses as though they were mental disorders which should be diminished or abolished if possible. The idea that emotional pain is a state which requires assessment, medical treatment or 'counselling' is dehumanizing. It is assuming that the best form of human life should always be one of happiness, and that that state can be brought about or its opposite removed, by some form of professional expertise and possibly medication. The promotion of this idea is arguably a harm to patients, their families, health care professionals and society in general.

Horwitz and Wakefield (quoted in Section 10.1) noted that although the DSM-IV criteria for diagnosis of a major depressive disorder have a clause to exclude the symptomatic bereaved from being diagnosed as having a major depressive disorder for the first two months after bereavement, in reality a longer period of intense but normal sadness may occur resulting in 10–20% of bereaved people being mistakenly diagnosed as having a major depressive illness. Labelling such patients with a psychiatric diagnosis, with the attendant treatment sequelae, may indeed be harmful.[56]

Experienced clinical workers have recognized that bereavement is a normal process and that bereaved people are not 'sick'. Parkes *et al.* note that 'Bereaved people who come to think of themselves as sick easily become dependent on those who adopt the role of therapist'.[57] They further comment that specialized counsellors for bereavement 'need to be aware of the dangers of medicalizing normal life crises'.

A second form of harm is the implication that ordinary people are not able to cope with the crises of their lives without professional assistance. This is profoundly patronizing and de-skilling for society; it treats ordinary people like children who need to be comforted by a representative of the 'Nanny State.' We have already noted that even writers enthusiastic about bereavement care agree that input from outside the family is neither necessary nor helpful to the majority of bereaved people.

Third, there is considerable potential for direct harm to relatives. Horwitz and Wakefield noted that 'Interventions such as grief counselling and efforts that force people to acknowledge their grief have not been shown to be very effective and can be harmful. Indeed, an alarmingly high number of grieving people worsen after receiving treatment'.[58] Bereavement counselling could itself be intrusive or exhausting—authors experienced in bereavement counselling describe seven dimensions of loss which should be covered in a single interview, and which, if not spontaneously mentioned by the client, should be explored by additional questions.[59]

Fourth, there is a harm to those working in end of life care. These same authors note the possibilities of burn-out in professionals who have unreasonable expectations of what they should achieve by psychological care of patients and their families.[60]

It is a matter of particular concern that the *End of life care strategy* has specified that bereavement care should be offered to, and be available for, all those who were close to the patient. In the publicly funded NHS where care has increasingly become target-focused, this expectation is enormous (and probably unrealistic), yet it is being placed on health care professionals who are likely to find it stressful and burdensome.

From the above evidence and arguments we must conclude that it is highly controversial whether those involved in end of life care should routinely assess those close to the patient for risk of morbid bereavement, and then offer a general bereavement follow-up service to all those who have sustained the loss.

10.3.iii Cost-effectiveness of benefit to relatives

Is the health-related benefit to relatives sufficient to justify the expenditure of resources? It is impossible to answer this question in the absence of research comparing the benefit to relatives with the benefits which patients would receive if those resources were devoted instead to their care.

There is some evidence of reduction in relatives' distress in terms of guilt, dependency, loss of control, despair, numbness, shock, and disbelief, when patients were cared for within a hospice programme.[61] Nevertheless, research is needed to evaluate the investment of staff time required to achieve this. In such research it would be necessary to distinguish between time invested by staff to assist the family to care for the patient, and time invested in attempting to reduce the distress of relatives where there is very little or no benefit to the patient, for example where the relatives are not caring for the patient. Time spent supporting family members in caring for the patient is clearly likely to result in indirect benefits to the patient, especially where those family carers shoulder a significant burden of care in the last months of the patient's life.

In the absence of evidence it is impossible to make a judgement about whether the health-related benefits to relatives could justify the expenditure of resources which are lost from patient care. However, since it is clear that time spent with relatives is lost to direct patient care it seems reasonable to argue that excessive time should not be spent with relatives. The resource of time must be rationed between relatives and patients. Where significant time is spent with relatives but the staff numbers are relatively low (as is likely in a publicly funded health care system), then either the staff will pay the price by working persistently more hours than is reasonable or funded, or patients will pay the price by having less than reasonable or adequate care.

10.4 **Conclusions**

1) The aims of end of life care should be: the relief of pain and other symptoms; restoration or maintenance of physical function; prolongation of life where the expected benefit outweighs the harms and risks and the patient wants the treatment; and the sensitive provision to patients of information about their illness in order to enable them to take part in decisions and lessen emotional distress. Coordinated care is required to meet nursing needs.

2) Whole person or holistic care is acceptable as an aim of end of life care, but the term must be used with caution (and humility) because a patient's wholeness extends well beyond anything that health care interventions at the end of life can encompass.

3) Whereas a special therapeutic relationship, founded on an implicit promise and associated with specific obligations, exists between professionals and patients, there is no therapeutic relationship between professionals and the relatives of patients.

4) There are obligations to relatives of a general nature: to provide information (subject to constraints of confidentiality); to offer advice on the care of the patient; to provide assistance with nursing care of the patient according to the patient's agreed care plan; to behave sensitively in the face of the inevitable family distress.

5) Pursuing the relatives' interests at the expense of the patient's health interests cannot be justified, and where the patient lacks capacity it is also likely to be deemed unlawful in terms of UK law.

6) The evidence which might support provision of a general bereavement service is at best inconclusive.

References

1. Medical Schools Council (2008). *The consensus statement on the role of the doctor* Available at http://www.medschools.ac.uk/documents/ FinalconsensusstatementontheRoleoftheDoctor.doc (accessed on 20.1.09).

2. British Medical Association (2007). *Withholding and withdrawing life-prolonging medical treatment*, 3rd edn. Blackwell, Oxford, p. 4.

3. World Health Organization (2002). *National cancer programmes: policies and managerial guidelines*, 2nd edn. WHO, Geneva.

4. Shakespeare W (*c.*1606). *Macbeth*. Act V, Scene 3.

5. Murray Parkes C, Relf M, Couldrick A (1996). *Counselling in terminal care and bereavement*. BPS Books, Leicester, p. 58.

6. Murray Parkes *et al.*, op. cit. (ref. 5), p. 65.

7. Heath I (2008). *Matters of life and death*. Radcliffe Publishing, Oxford, p. 41.

8. Department of Health (2008). *End of life care strategy*. DoH, London, p. 82.

9. Horwitz A, Wakefield J (2007). *Loss of sadness: how psychiatry transformed normal sorrow into depressive disorder*. Oxford University Press, Oxford.

10. American Psychiatric Association (2000). *Diagnostic and statistical manual of mental disorders*, 4th edn, revised. APA, Washington, DC.

11. Horwitz, Wakefield, op. cit. (ref. 9), p. 6.

12. Horwitz, Wakefield, op. cit. (ref. 9), pp. 27–8.

13. Horwitz, Wakefield, op. cit. (ref. 9), p. 6.

14. Cancer Action Team (2007). *Holistic common assessment of supportive and palliative care needs for adults with cancer: assessment guidance*. Cancer Action Team, London, pp. 13–14.

15. Friedman T (2008). Current provision of psychosocial care within palliative care. In Lloyd-Williams M (ed.), *Psychosocial issues in palliative care*, 2nd edn. Oxford University Press, Oxford, p. 109.

16. Timonen M, Liukkonen T (2008). Management of depression in adults. *BMJ* **336**:435–9.

17. Lloyd-Williams M, Reeve J, Kissane D (2008). Distress in palliative care patients: developing patient-centred approaches to clinical management. *European Journal of Cancer* **44**:1133–8.

18. Pessin H, Evcimen YA, Apostolatos AJ, Breitbart W (2008). Diagnosis, assessment, and treatment of depression in palliative care. In *Psychosocial issues in palliative care* (ref. 15), p. 132.

19. Horwitz, Wakefield, op. cit. (ref. 9), p. 147.

20. O'Keefe N, Ranjith G (2007). Depression, demoralisation or adjustment disorder? Understanding emotional distress in the severely medically ill. *Clin Med* **7**:478–81.

21. Horwitz, Wakefield, op. cit. (ref. 9), p. 148.

22. Passik SD, Kirsh KL, Lloyd-Williams M (2008). Anxiety and adjustment disorders. In *Psychosocial issues in palliative care* (ref. 15), pp. 115, 122–3.

23. Pessin H, Evcimen YA, Apostolatos J, Breitbart W (2008). Diagnosis, assessment, and treatment of depression in palliative care. In *Psychosocial issues in palliative care* (ref. 15), p. 137.

24. Horwitz A, Wakefield J, op. cit. (ref. 9), p. 142.

25. Pessin H, Evcimen YA, Apostolatos AJ, Breitbart W (2008). Diagnosis, assessment, and treatment of depression in palliative care. In *Psychosocial issues in palliative care* (ref. 15), p. 129.

26. Horwitz, Wakefield, op. cit. (ref. 9), pp. 155–156.

27. Middleton H, Shaw I, Hull S, Feder G (2005). NICE guidelines on the management of depression. *BMJ* **330**:267.

28. Parker G (2007). Is depression overdiagnosed? *BMJ* **335**:328.

29. Turner EH, Rosenthal R (2008). Efficacy of antidepressants. *BMJ* **336**:516–7.

30. O'Keefe, Ranjith, op. cit. (ref. 20), p. 481.

31. Cathcart F (2006). Psychological distress in patients with advanced cancer. *Clin Med* **6**:148–50.

32. Heath, op. cit. (ref. 7), pp. 58–69.

33. Heath, op. cit. (ref. 7), p. 45.

34. Randall F, Downie RS (2006). *The philosophy of palliative care: critique and reconstruction*. Oxford University Press, Oxford, pp. 25–51.

35. World Health Organization (2004). *Palliative care: the solid facts*. WHO, Geneva, p. 9, 18.

36. Attwood C (2008). Spiritual care at the end of life. *Inside Palliative Care* **6**:16–17.

37. Heath, op. cit. (ref. 7), pp. 34–5.

38. Marvell A [1650] (1972). An Horation Ode upon Cromwell's return from Ireland. In Gardner H (ed.), *The new Oxford book of English verse*. Clarendon Press, Oxford, pp. 329–33.

39. International Labour Organization (2008). *International standard classification of occupations (ISCO), draft ISCO-08 Group definitions occupations in health*. ILO, Geneva.

40. Franks PJ, *et al.* (2000). The level of need for palliative care: a systematic review of the literature. *Palliative Medicine* **14**:98.

41. Department of Health, op. cit. (ref. 8), pp. 113, 108, 107.

42. Panke JT, Ferrell BR (2004). Emotional problems in the family. In *Oxford textbook of palliative medicine*, 3rd edn. Oxford University Press, Oxford, p. 986.

43. Kissane D (2004). Bereavement. In *Oxford textbook of palliative medicine* (ref. 42), p. 1137.

44. Brewin T (1996). *The friendly professional*. Eurocommunica Publications, Bognor Regis, pp. 74–9.

45. Finlay I (2006). Crossing the "bright line"—difficult decisions at the end of life. *Clin Med* **6**:398–402.

46. World Health Organization (2004). *Better palliative care for older people*. WHO, Geneva, p. 29.

47. National Institute for Clinical Excellence (2004). *Improving supportive and palliative care for adults with cancer*. NICE, London, p. 158–166.

48. Department of Health, op. cit. (ref. 8), p. 109.

49. Department of Health, op. cit. (ref. 8), p. 112.

50. Horwitz, Wakefield, op. cit. (ref. 9), p. 33.

51. World Health Organization (2002). *National cancer control programmes: policies and managerial guidelines*, 2nd edn. WHO, Geneva.

52. Hawton K (2007). Complicated grief after bereavement. *BMJ* **334**:962–3.

53. Parkes CM, Relf M, Couldrick A (1996). *Counselling in terminal care and bereavement*. BPS Books, Leicester, p. 106.

54. Hawton, op. cit. (ref. 52), p. 962.

55. Kissane D (2004). Bereavement. In *Oxford textbook of palliative medicine* (ref. 42), p. 1142.

56. Horwitz, Wakefield, op. cit. (ref. 9), p. 32.

57. Parkes *et al.*, op. cit. (ref. 53), p. 47.

58. Horwitz, Wakefield, op. cit. (ref. 9), p. 33.

59. Parkes *et al.*, op. cit. (ref. 53), p. 147.

60. Parkes *et al.*, op. cit. (ref. 53), p. 46.

61. Panke, Ferrell, op. cit. (ref. 42), p. 989.

General conclusions

The philosophy of medicine and of end of life care in particular which emerged in the second half of the twentieth century stressed the importance of patient choice in the light of information provided by the doctor. In particular, doctors supported patients:

- by ascertaining how much information patients required and providing it sensitively;
- by listening to patients' views about their own goals and values;
- by discussing the possible impact of various treatments on their lives so as to work out which treatment would benefit a particular patient;
- by giving explanations and advice based on professional experience.

The patient choice emerging from discussions of this kind could be seen as reflecting both the patient's goals and values and the doctor's medical responsibilities and expertise. It was in fact joint decision-making directed at the best interests of the patient. Those 'best interests' could be spelled out in terms of the prolongation of life, the relief of suffering and the maintenance of function. It would be wrong to suggest that consultations with this content in end of life care were inhumane or 'medicalized'. There is no reason to think that the professionals in attendance would be other than caring, compassionate or friendly. But it must be stressed that being caring, compassionate and friendly are not matters of expertise. When Dame Cicely Saunders suggested that professionals should 'watch and listen' she was not recommending a technical intervention. She was thinking simply of the invaluable comfort which one human being can give to another facing life's end.

To a great extent professional bodies are losing sight of these simplicities. Consumerism is taking over health care, and the best interests of patients are being seen as patients getting whatever it is they choose, in terms of treatments, care and place of death. If this is a cultural change then it will continue whether we like it or not. Currently politicians believe that patients want choice above all, and professionals have not effectively opposed them, so we can expect many politically driven initiatives such as performance measures based mainly or solely on achievement of patients' choices. There is a real possibility that health care professionals become merely the unwitting instruments of politicians. Certain cautions should be mentioned, in ascending order of importance.

Politicians have long been looking for sticks (performance measures such as quality markers, targets, 'metrics') to beat the backs of those providing end of life care. They obviously cannot use waiting times, but preferred place of death is an obvious candidate. So we can expect pressure on patients to choose in advance what is likely to be achieved, or urgent transfer of imminently dying patients to their previously chosen place of death, just to achieve a satisfactory performance rating for the professional or service.

Second (and especially relevant in the UK), it is logically impossible to run a consumerist choice health service within a publicly funded health service. We outlined the key concepts of the free market economy in Chapter 1 (competition, prevention from harm, worldwide alternatives, consumer responsibility for what is chosen, consumer payment for what is chosen). The consumerist choice model entitles and coerces patients at the end of life to choose from the entire range of technically possible treatments and care, and then forces them to confront sufficient information to take consumer responsibility for their choices. A service run on these lines is incompatible with a service, such as the National Health Service, which is free at the point of delivery, in which the values of equity and cost-effectiveness are essential, and where professionals still take some responsibility for treatment decisions. Many people may prefer an end of life service run on free market lines; our point is simply that it is producing confusion when it is introduced into a publicly funded health service.

Finally, it is a belittling view of human nature to think that what matters most to human beings facing life's last mystery is consumer choice, especially of where to die. This view devalues and diminishes what patients, their families and professionals can achieve together.

In conclusion we wish to suggest that an end of life service should have the following characteristics:

1 **Realism.** It should not claim that it can diagnose, treat and resolve every problem—physical, emotional, social, and spiritual—of patients approaching the ends of their lives, far less those of their families.

2 **Fairness.** Priority in care should be directed at patients, not at patients and families equally; cost-effectiveness considerations justifiably limit availability of very expensive life-prolonging treatments and ways of delivering care when publicly funded; the scarce resource of specialist palliative care should be allocated according to complexity of patient need, not patient choice; telephone advice from specialist palliative care and educational programmes should be available to all health care professionals.

3 **Humanity.** Very ill patients should not be subjected to intrusive interviews or 'assessment tools'. Instead, professionals should listen to patients and be able to converse with them in a friendly manner on the issues of life and death, while working jointly with patients in decisions about their treatment and care. This requires time, maturity of character, and experience rather than course-based training.

4 **Adoptability.** With realistic and modest characteristics such as these, end of life care of a good quality can be provided equitably in all settings.

Index